CONTENTS

SNACK & DESSERT RECIPES 97

INTRODUCTION

What is the Hamilton Beach Indoor MultiGrill ?

The Hamilton Beach Indoor MultiGrill has a large surface to cook on – 100 square inch, to be precise. So, cooking for a crowd is a breeze with this appliance. Being able to prepare a decent amount of food in a very short time makes this indoor grill incredibly appealing. And the fact that your meat will not stick to it is an added plus. You can simply arrange your food onto the bottom plate, lower the lid, and cut the cooking time in half without having to flip over your ingredients. It has three cooking modes of the Grill Mode – Allows you to cook your meats perfectly and the Griddle Mode – Is perfect for your eggs and morning pancakes the Bacon Mode – Will help you get the crispiest strips of bacon ever.

How to Using the Hamilton Beach 3-in-1 MultiGrill?

Being a three-in-one kind of appliance may trick you into thinking that this grill is overwhelming to use, but once you plug it in and start cooking, you will see that it is not only very straightforward, but it also doesn't require particular grilling skills, either.

Just follow our step-by-step instructions, and you're good to go.

Grilling

First of all, make sure always to use oven mittens for safety and protection when grilling. Start by aligning the tabs of the grill plates with their openings. Press well until you hear the clicking sound, which indicates that everything is into place. The drip tray should be slided in.

1.Plug the device in. The red indicator light should be on.

2.Set the desired temperature (250 to 400 degrees F) to preheat the grill.

3.When preheated, the green indicator light will turn on. At this point, you can place the food onto the plate for grilling.

4.Depending on the method of cooking, you may lower the grill lid if desired.

5. Lift the lid halfway through to check the food. If done, transfer to a plate.

6.Unplug the device and let it cool completely before cleaning the grill. Make sure not to touch the tray until it is completely cool.

Using the Griddle

Just like with grilling, it is highly recommended you use oven mittens when using the griddle, as well.

1.Plug the device in and make sure that the drip tray is in place. If you need a larger cooking surface, open the unit. Keep in mind, though, that that will require more time to cook and turning the food over halfway through.

2.Adjust the preferred temperature and wait for the green light to turn on.

3.When preheated, open the locked hinge as far as it goes, and lay it on your working surface.

4.Arrange the food on top of the griddle and start cooking.

5.Halfway through, flip over to ensure even cooking.

6.Transfer to a plate and unplug the appliance. Wait until it is completely cool to clean, and do not touch until cool enough to handle.

Cooking Bacon

If you depend on your crispy bacon for breakfast, then cooking it on the HB 3-in-1 grill will be your go-to method.

1.First, you will need to make sure that the kickstand is in position, as it is important for draining the bacon grease away. You can do this by lifting the back of the unit and rotating the kickstand. That should put it in place.

2.Plug the unit in.

3.For best (and crispiest) results, preheat the grill to 400 degrees F, keeping the unit closed in the meantime. Wait for the green indicator light to turn on.

4.Once preheated, open the lid and arrange the bacon onto the bottom plate.

5.Lower the lid and let the bacon cook. Normal bacon slices usually take between 7 to 10 minutes to become super crispy. You can cook it with the lid open as well, but keep in mind that keeping it closed will allow splatter-free cooking and even crispiness.

6.Once the desired doneness is reached, lift the cover and grab some plastic utensils to transfer the bacon to a serving plate.

7.Unplug the grill and let it sit until cool enough to handle. Do not try to clean until completely cool.

Tips and tricks on cleaning the appliance

Before you even attempt to clean the appliance, make sure that you:

Unplug the appliance first

Wait until the grill is completely safe to handle

Never immerse the cord, base, and plug into liquid

Never clean with abrasive cleaners

Do not use metal utensils as they can seriously damage the nonstick coat on the surface

Once you make sure that you handle with safety and caution, follow these steps:

1.Unplug the device.

2.Push the button that releases the upper plate of the grill. Remove it and set aside. Do the same with the bottom plate. Press release and set it aside.

3.Check the condition of the grill. Sometimes grease finds its way under the top and bottom plates. If not completely clean, grab a soapy sponge and gently wipe the surface. Then, with a damp cloth, wipe again. Grab a clean towel (or kitchen towels) and pat dry.

4.Clean the outside of the unit, as well. Simply wipe with a damp cloth and then wipe it dry afterward.

5.Now, it is time to tackle the actual plates. You can clean them with a soft sponge drenched in warm, soapy water. Rinse under clean water, and then let dry completely before locking them back into place. And if this sounds easy, wait until you hear that they are all dishwasher safe. If you have a dishwashing machine in your kitchen, you can simply pop them in, and voila.

Troubleshooting and Fixing Common Issues

Although this is truly a unit of high quality, we shouldn't forget that there is nothing magical about it. It is an electric appliance, after all, and just like with any devices, when using the HB indoor grill, you may bump into some obstacles occasionally. But don't fret! We have compiled this section to make your life easier. Below, you will find the common issues users face when handling this indoor grill, and learn how to fix them, easily. The Device Won't Start. Check if the grill is actually plugged in. If it is but still cannot start, check your power outlet - maybe the issue is not in the unit at all. You can also check the breaker box to make sure power is working.

Remember, when plugged in, the indicator light will turn on.

The Grease Is Not Draining. If you have grease dripping, and not draining, there are two possible reasons for it. The first one is that your kickstand is not locked in place. Grab some oven mittens and check if it is sitting correctly – reassemble if needed. The second reason may occur if you haven't cleaned under the plates for some time. If not maintained regularly, the drain hole may get clogged. Unplug the unit and let cool completely, then clean around the drain hole well, to get rid of leftover gunk. The Grill Overcooks. If your food is overcooked, then it is not the grill's fault at all. Try to lower the temperature or cut the cooking time shorter. For meat, you can invest in a good thermostat that will measure the internal temperature so you can know precisely when the food is cooked. The Grill Undercooks. If your food is undercooked, obviously, the reason can be not enough cooking time or temperature. Try to cook longer and increase the heat if that is the issue. However, the grill can undercook your food if the plates are not placed correctly. Check the top and bottom plate and see if they are pressed into place. For best results, allow the grill to fully preheat before adding food to it, and cook with the lid lowered.

APPETIZER & SIDE DISHES

Lemony Green Beans

Servings: 3
Cooking Time: 6 Minutes

Ingredients:

- 2 tablespoons canola oil
- 2 garlic cloves, crushed
- 1 teaspoon red chili powder
- Salt, as required
- 1 pound fresh asparagus, trimmed

Directions:

1. In a bowl, place all ingredients except for lemon juice and toss to coat well.
2. Place the water tray in the bottom of Hamilton Beach Grill.
3. Place about 2 cups of lukewarm water into the water tray.
4. Place the drip pan over water tray and then arrange the heating element.
5. Now, place the grilling pan over heating element.
6. Plugin the Hamilton Beach Grill and press the 'Power' button to turn it on.
7. Then press 'Fan" button.
8. Set the temperature settings according to manufacturer's directions.
9. Cover the grill with lid and let it preheat.
10. After preheating, remove the lid and grease the grilling pan.
11. Place the asparagus over the grilling pan.
12. Cover with the lid and cook for about 5-6 minutes, turning occasionally.
13. Transfer the green beans into a bowl and drizzle with lemon juice.
14. Serve hot.

Nutrition Info: (Per Serving):Calories 118 ;Total Fat 9.7 g ;Saturated Fat 0.8 g ;Cholesterol 0mg ;Sodium 63 mg ;Total Carbs 7 g ;Fiber 3.5 g ;Sugar 2.9 g ;Protein 3.6 g

Grilled Butternut Squash

Servings: 4

Cooking Time: 8 Minutes

Ingredients:

- 1 medium butternut squash, sliced
- 1 tablespoon olive oil
- 1 ½ teaspoons dried oregano
- 1 teaspoon dried thyme
- 1/2 teaspoon salt
- 1/4 teaspoon black pepper

Directions:

1. Peel and slice the squash into ½ inch thick slices.
2. Remove the center of the slices to discard the seeds.
3. Toss the squash slices with remaining ingredients in a bowl.
4. Turn the "Selector" knob to the "Grill Panini" side.
5. Preheat the bottom grill of Hamilton Beach Grill at 350 degrees F and the upper grill plate on medium heat.
6. Once it is preheated, open the lid and place the squash in the Griddler.
7. Close the griddler's lid and grill the squash for 8 minutes.
8. Serve warm.

Nutrition Info: (Per Serving): Calories 249 ;Total Fat 11.9 g ;Saturated Fat 1.7 g ;Cholesterol 78 mg ;Sodium 79 mg ;Total Carbs 41.8 g ;Fiber 1.1 g ;Sugar 20.3 g ;Protein 15 g

Tarragon Asparagus

Servings: 4

Cooking Time: 4 Minutes

Ingredients:

- 2 lbs. fresh asparagus, trimmed
- 2 tablespoons olive oil
- 1 teaspoon salt
- 1/2 teaspoon black pepper
- 1/4 cup honey
- 4 tablespoons fresh tarragon, minced

Directions:

1. Liberally season the asparagus by tossing with oil, salt, pepper, honey, and tarragon.
2. Turn the "Selector" knob to the "Grill Panini" side.
3. Preheat the bottom grill of Hamilton Beach Grill at 300 degrees F and the upper grill plate on medium heat.
4. Once it is preheated, open the lid and place the asparagus in the Griddler.
5. Close the griddler's lid and grill the asparagus for 4 minutes.
6. Serve warm.

Nutrition Info: (Per Serving): Calories 148 ;Total Fat 15.7 g ;Saturated Fat 2.7 g ;Cholesterol 75 mg ;Sodium 94 mg ;Total Carbs 3.4 g ;Fiber 0.6 g ;Sugar 15 g ;Protein 14.1 g

Balsamic-glazed Carrots

Servings: 10

Cooking Time: 6 Minutes

Ingredients:

- 2 pounds Carrots, boiled for 3-4 minutes
- 3 tbsp Balsamic Vinegar
- 1 tsp ground Ginger
- 1 tsp Thyme
- 1 ½ tbsp Maple Syrup
- ½ tbsp Lime Juice
- Salt and Pepper, to taste

Directions:

1. Preheat your grill to 400 degrees F.
2. Meanwhile, cut the carrots in half lengthwise.
3. Place the remaining ingredients in a bowl and whisk well to combine.
4. Brush the carrots with the mixture, on all sides.
5. When the green light is on, open the grill and spray with some cooking spray.
6. Arrange the carrots on top of the bottom plate and cook for 3 minutes.
7. Flip over and cook for 3 more minutes on the other side.
8. Serve and enjoy!

Nutrition Info: Calories 50 ;Total Fats 1g ;Carbs 12g ;Protein 1g ;Fiber: 3g

Cauliflower Steaks

Servings: 4

Cooking Time: 9 Minutes

Ingredients:

- 2 large heads cauliflower
- ¼ cup olive oil
- ½ teaspoons garlic powder
- ½ teaspoons paprika
- Kosher salt, to taste
- Black pepper, to taste
- 2 cups cheddar cheese, shredded
- Ranch dressing, for drizzling
- 8 cooked bacon slices, crumbled
- 2 tablespoons chives, chopped

Directions:

1. Mix olive oil, garlic powder, paprika, salt, and black pepper in a bowl
2. Slice the cauliflower into ¾ inch thick steaks and rub them with the olive oil mixture.
3. Turn the "Selector" knob to the "Grill Panini" side.
4. Preheat the bottom grill of Hamilton Beach Grill at 350 degrees F and the upper grill plate on medium heat.
5. Once it is preheated, open the lid and place the cauliflower steaks in the Griddler.
6. Close the griddler's lid and grill the steaks for 8 minutes until lightly charred.
7. Open the lid and drizzle bacon, cheddar cheese, ranch dressing and chives on top.
8. Cook for 1 minute until the cheese is melted.
9. Serve warm.

Nutrition Info: (Per Serving): Calories 278 ;Total Fat 3.8 g ;Saturated Fat 0.7 g ;Cholesterol 2 mg ;Sodium 620 mg ;Total Carbs 13.3 g ;Fiber 2.4 g ;Sugar 1.2 g ;Protein 5.4 g

Brussel Sprout Skewers

Servings: 8
Cooking Time: 7 Minutes

Ingredients:

- 24 Brussel Sprouts
- 2 tbsp Balsamic Glaze
- 4 tbsp Olive Oil
- ½ tsp Garlic Powder
- Salt and Pepper, to taste

Directions:

1. Preheat your grill to 375 degrees F.
2. In the meantime, trim the brussel sprouts and cut the in half.
3. Thread onto soaked wooden or metal skewers.
4. Drizzle with olive oil and sprinkle with the seasonings.
5. Place onto the bottom plate and cook uncovered for 4 minutes.
6. Turn over and cook for another 3 minutes or so.
7. Serve as desired and enjoy!

Nutrition Info: Calories 92 ;Total Fats 6g ;Carbs 6g ;Protein 1g ;Fiber: 2g

Shrimp With Dipping Sauce

Servings: 6

Cooking Time: 4 Minutes

Ingredients:

- 1½ pounds jumbo shrimp, peeled, deveined, and patted dry
- 2 teaspoons canola oil
- ¼ teaspoon paprika
- Salt and ground black pepper, as required
- ¼ cup warm jalapeño jelly
- ¼ cup chili sauce

Directions:

1. Brush the shrimp with oil lightly and then sprinkle with paprika, salt and black pepper.
2. Place the water tray in the bottom of Hamilton Beach Grill.
3. Place about 2 cups of lukewarm water into the water tray.
4. Place the drip pan over water tray and then, arrange the heating element.
5. Now, place the grilling pan over heating element.
6. Plugin the Hamilton Beach Grill and press the 'Power' button to turn it on.
7. Then press 'Fan" button.
8. Set the temperature settings according to manufacturer's directions.
9. Cover the grill with lid and let it preheat.
10. After preheating, remove the lid and grease the grilling pan.
11. Place the shrimp over the grilling pan.
12. Cover with the lid and cook for about 2 minutes per side.
13. Meanwhile, in a bowl, place jalapeño jelly and chili sauce and mix well.
14. Serve warm shrimp with dipping sauce.

Nutrition Info: (Per Serving):Calories 167 ;Total Fat 3.5 g ;Saturated Fat 0.7 g ;Cholesterol 239 mg ;Sodium 584 mg ;Total Carbs 6.6 g ;Fiber 0.1 g ;Sugar 4.1 g ;Protein 25.9 g

Grilled Brussels Sprouts

Servings: 2

Cooking Time: 9 Minutes

Ingredients:

- 1 lb. brussels sprouts, halved
- 3 tablespoons olive oil
- ¼ cup balsamic vinegar
- 1 tablespoon honey
- 1 tablespoon mustard
- 2 teaspoons crushed red pepper flakes
- Kosher salt
- ½ cup Parmesan, grated

Directions:

1. Mix oil, vinegar, honey, mustard, red pepper flakes, and salt in a bowl.
2. Toss in brussels sprout and toss well to coat.
3. Turn the "Selector" knob to the "Grill Panini" side.
4. Preheat the bottom grill of Hamilton Beach Grill at 350 degrees F and the upper grill plate on medium heat.
5. Once it is preheated, open the lid and place the brussels sprouts in the Griddler.
6. Close the griddler's lid and grill the brussels sprouts for 7-9 minutes until lightly charred.
7. Garnish with parmesan.

Nutrition Info: (Per Serving): Calories 121 ;Total Fat 3.8 g ;Saturated Fat 0.7 g ;Cholesterol 22 mg ;Sodium 620 mg ;Total Carbs 8.3 g ;Fiber 2.4 g ;Sugar 1.2 g ;Protein 5.4 g

Grilled And Dressed Romaine Head

Servings: 4
Cooking Time: 5 Minutes

Ingredients:

- 2 Hearts of Romaine
- ½ cup Olive Oil
- 2 Eg Yolks
- 2 Whole Garlic Cloves
- ½ tsp Dijon Mustard
- 2 Anchovies
- 3 tbsp Parmesan Cheese
- 4 tbsp Lemon Juice
- Salt an Pepper, to taste

Directions:

1. Preheat your grill to medium high.
2. Place all of the dressing ingredients to the bowl of your food processor.
3. Pulse until smooth and set aside.
4. When the grill is ready, open the lid and spray with some cooking spray.
5. Place the romaine heart onto the bottom plate and cook for 3 minutes.
6. Flip over and cook for 2 more minutes.
7. Arrange on a large serving plate.
8. Drizzle with the dressing.
9. Enjoy!

Nutrition Info: Calories 88 ;Total Fats 4g ;Carbs 3g ;Protein 2.5g ;Fiber: 0.4g

Balsamic Bell Peppers

Servings: 4
Cooking Time: 10 Minutes

Ingredients:

- 1 pound small bell peppers, halved and seeded
- 1 tablespoon olive oil
- Salt and ground black pepper, as required
- 1 tablespoon balsamic vinegar

Directions:

1. Brush the bell pepper halves with oil and then sprinkle with salt and pepper.
2. Place the water tray in the bottom of Hamilton Beach Grill.
3. Place about 2 cups of lukewarm water into the water tray.
4. Place the drip pan over water tray and then arrange the heating element.
5. Now, place the grilling pan over heating element.
6. Plugin the Hamilton Beach Grill and press the 'Power' button to turn it on.
7. Then press 'Fan" button.
8. Set the temperature settings according to manufacturer's directions.
9. Cover the grill with lid and let it preheat.
10. After preheating, remove the lid and grease the grilling pan.
11. Place the bell pepper halves over the grilling pan.
12. Cover with the lid and cook for about 8-10 minutes, flipping once halfway through.
13. Transfer the bell pepper halves onto a plate and drizzle with vinegar.
14. Serve immediately.

Nutrition Info: (Per Serving):Calories 40 ;Total Fat 3.6 g ;Saturated Fat 0.5 g ;Cholesterol 0mg ;Sodium 40 mg ;Total Carbs 2.3 g ;Fiber 0.4 g ;Sugar 1.5 g ;Protein 0.3 g

Grilled Eggplant

Servings: 4
Cooking Time: 8 Minutes

Ingredients:

- 2 small eggplants, half-inch slices
- 1/4 cup olive oil
- 2 tablespoons lime juice
- 3 teaspoons Cajun seasoning

Directions:

1. Liberally season the eggplant slices with oil, lemon juice, and Cajun seasoning.
2. Turn the "Selector" knob to the "Grill Panini" side.
3. Preheat the bottom grill of Hamilton Beach Grill at 300 degrees F and the upper grill plate on medium heat.
4. Once it is preheated, open the lid and place the eggplant slices in the Griddler.
5. Close the griddler's lid and grill the eggplant for 8 minutes until slightly charred.
6. Serve warm.

Nutrition Info: (Per Serving): Calories 172 ;Total Fat 11.1 g ;Saturated Fat 5.8 g ;Cholesterol 610 mg ;Sodium 749 mg ;Total Carbs 16.9 g ;Fiber 0.2 g ;Sugar 0.2 g ;Protein 3.5 g

Butter Glazed Green Beans

Servings: 4

Cooking Time: 5 Minutes

Ingredients:

- 1-lb. fresh green beans, trimmed
- 1/2 teaspoon Cajun seasoning
- 1 tablespoon butter, melted

Directions:

1. Toss green beans with butter and Cajun seasoning in a bowl.
2. Turn the "Selector" knob to the "Grill Panini" side.
3. Preheat the bottom grill of Hamilton Beach Grill at 350 degrees F and the upper grill plate on medium heat.
4. Once it is preheated, open the lid and place the green beans in the Griddler.
5. Close the griddler's lid and grill the green beans for 5 minutes.
6. Serve warm.

Nutrition Info: (Per Serving): Calories 304 ;Total Fat 30.6 g ;Saturated Fat 13.1 g ;Cholesterol 131 mg ;Sodium 834 mg ;Total Carbs 21.4 g ;Fiber 0.2 g ;Sugar 0.3 g ;Protein 4.6 g

Parmesan Zucchini

Servings: 4

Cooking Time: 7 Minutes

Ingredients:

- 3 medium zucchinis, cut into ½-inch slices
- 2 tablespoons extra-virgin olive oil
- Salt and ground black pepper, as required
- ¼ cup parmesan cheese, shredded

Directions:

1. Brush the zucchini slices with oil and then sprinkle with salt and pepper.
2. Place the water tray in the bottom of Hamilton Beach Grill.
3. Place about 2 cups of lukewarm water into the water tray.
4. Place the drip pan over water tray and then arrange the heating element.
5. Now, place the grilling pan over heating element.
6. Plugin the Hamilton Beach Grill and press the 'Power' button to turn it on.
7. Then press 'Fan" button.
8. Set the temperature settings according to manufacturer's directions.
9. Cover the grill with lid and let it preheat.
10. After preheating, remove the lid and grease the grilling pan.
11. Place the zucchini slices over the grilling pan.
12. Cover with the lid and cook for about 5-7 minutes, flipping once halfway through.
13. Transfer the zucchini slices onto a plate and sprinkle with cheese.
14. Serve immediately.

Nutrition Info: (Per Serving):Calories 104 ;Total Fat 8.6 g ;Saturated Fat 1.9 g ;Cholesterol 4 mg ;Sodium 138 mg ;Total Carbs 5.1 g ;Fiber 1.6 g ;Sugar 2.5 g ;Protein 3.7 g

Cauliflower Zucchini Skewers

Servings: 8

Cooking Time: 10 Minutes

Ingredients:

- 4 large zucchinis sliced
- 1 head cauliflower, cut into florets
- Olive oil, for drizzling
- kosher salt, to taste
- Black pepper, to taste
- 1/4 cup crumbled feta

Directions:

1. Alternately, thread the cauliflower and zucchini slices on the wooden skewers.
2. Drizzle olive oil, black pepper and salt over the skewers.
3. Turn the "Selector" knob to the "Grill Panini" side.
4. Preheat the bottom grill of Hamilton Beach Grill at 300 degrees F and the upper grill plate on medium heat.
5. Once it is preheated, open the lid and place the skewers in the Griddler.
6. Close the griddler's lid and grill the cauliflower skewers for 10 minutes.
7. Garnish with feta cheese.
8. Serve.

Nutrition Info: (Per Serving): Calories 191 ;Total Fat 12.2 g ;Saturated Fat 2.4 g ;Cholesterol 110 mg ;Sodium 276 mg ;Total Carbs 5 g ;Fiber 0.9 g ;Sugar 1.4 g ;Protein 8.8 g

Grilled Zucchini

Servings: 4

Cooking Time: 6 Minutes

Ingredients:

- 1-pound Zucchini
- 1 tbsp Lemon Juice
- 2 Garlic Cloves, minced
- 2 tbsp Olive Oil
- 1 tsp Italian Seasoning
- Salt and Pepper, to taste

Directions:

1. Trim and peel the zucchini. Cut into thick slices and place in a bowl.
2. Add all of the remaining ingredients and mix well so that the zucchini slices are completely coated.
3. Cover the bowl and place in the fridge for about one hour.
4. Menawhile, preheat your HB grill to 375 degrees F.
5. When the green light turns on, open the grill and place the zucchini slices onto the bottom plate.
6. Cook with the lid off, for three minutes. Flip over and cook for another three minutes.
7. Serve as desired and enjoy!

Nutrition Info: Calories 76 ;Total Fats 7g ;Carbs 1g ;Protein 0g ;Fiber: 0g

Garlicky Mushroom Skewers With Balsamic Vinegar

Servings: 4

Cooking Time: 4 Minutes

Ingredients:

- 2 pounds Button Mushrooms, halved
- 1 tbsp Tamari Sauce
- 2 tbsp Balsamic Vinegar
- ½ tsp Dried Thyme
- 2 large Garlic Cloves, minced
- Salt and Pepper, to taste

Directions:

1. Place the tamari, balsamic, thyme, and garlic, in a bowl.
2. Season with some salt and pepper and mix well to combine.
3. Add the mushrooms and toss to coat them well.
4. Cover the bowl and place in the fridge for about 30 minutes.
5. While the mushrooms are marinating, soak your wooden skewers in water to prevent burning.
6. Preheat your grill to 375 degrees F.
7. Thread the mushrooms onto your skewers and place on top of the bottom plate.
8. Grill for 2 minutes, then flip over, and grill for another two minutes, or until tender.
9. Serve and enjoy!

Nutrition Info: Calories 62 ;Total Fats 1g ;Carbs 9g ;Protein 7g ;Fiber: 2g

Simple Mushrooms

Servings: 2

Cooking Time: 5 Minutes

Ingredients:

- 8 ounces shiitake mushrooms, stems discarded
- 1 tablespoon vegetable oil
- 1 garlic clove, minced
- Salt and ground black pepper, as required

Directions:

1. In a bowl, place all ingredients and toss to coat well.
2. Place the water tray in the bottom of Hamilton Beach Grill.
3. Place about 2 cups of lukewarm water into the water tray.
4. Place the drip pan over water tray and then arrange the heating element.
5. Now, place the grilling pan over heating element.
6. Plugin the Hamilton Beach Grill and press the 'Power' button to turn it on.
7. Then press 'Fan" button.
8. Set the temperature settings according to manufacturer's directions.
9. Cover the grill with lid and let it preheat.
10. After preheating, remove the lid and grease the grilling pan.
11. Place the mushrooms over the grilling pan.
12. Cover with the lid and cook for about 4-5 minutes, turning occasionally.
13. Serve hot.

Nutrition Info: (Per Serving):Calories 87 ;Total Fat 7.1 g ;Saturated Fat 1.3 g ;Cholesterol 0 mg ;Sodium 84 mg ;Total Carbs 4.2 g ;Fiber 1.2 g ;Sugar 2 g ;Protein 3.7 g

Grilled Veggies With Vinaigrette

Servings: 4
Cooking Time: 7 Minutes

Ingredients:

- Vinaigrette:
- 1/4 cup red wine vinegar
- 1 tablespoon Dijon mustard
- 1 tablespoon honey
- 1/2 teaspoon salt
- 1/8 teaspoon pepper
- 1/4 cup canola oil
- 1/4 cup olive oil
- Vegetables:
- 2 large sweet onions, sliced
- 2 yellow summer squash, sliced
- 2 large red peppers, seeded and sliced

Directions:

1. Whisk wine vinegar, Dijon mustard, honey, salt, black pepper olive oil and canola oil in a bowl.
2. Turn the "Selector" knob to the "Grill Panini" side.
3. Preheat the bottom grill of Hamilton Beach Grill at 350 degrees F and the upper grill plate on medium heat.
4. Once it is preheated, open the lid and place the vegetable slices in the Griddler.
5. Close the griddler's lid and grill the onions and peppers for 5 minutes and summer squash for 7 minutes.
6. Transfer the veggies to a serving plate and drizzle the vinaigrette on top.
7. Serve warm.

Nutrition Info: (Per Serving): Calories 341 ;Total Fat 4 g ;Saturated Fat 0.5 g ;Cholesterol 69 mg ;Sodium 547 mg ;Total Carbs 6.4 g ;Fiber 1.2 g ;Sugar 1 g ;Protein 10.3 g

Grilled Mushroom Skewers

Servings: 6
Cooking Time: 3 Minutes

Ingredients:

- 2 pounds mushrooms, sliced
- 2 tablespoons balsamic vinegar
- 1 tablespoon soy sauce
- 3 garlic cloves, chopped
- 1/2 teaspoon thyme, chopped
- Salt and black pepper to taste

Directions:

1. Toss mushrooms with balsamic vinegar, soy sauce, garlic, thyme, black pepper and salt in a bowl.
2. Thread the mushroom slices on mini wooden skewers.
3. Turn the "Selector" knob to the "Grill Panini" side.
4. Preheat the bottom grill of Hamilton Beach Grill at 350 degrees F and the upper grill plate on medium heat.
5. Once it is preheated, open the lid and place mushroom skewers horizontally in the Griddler.
6. Close the griddler's lid and grill the mushrooms for 3 minutes.
7. Serve warm.

Nutrition Info: (Per Serving): Calories 418 ;Total Fat 15.7 g ;Saturated Fat 2.7 g ;Cholesterol 75 mg ;Sodium 94 mg ;Total Carbs 10.4 g ;Fiber 0.1 g ;Sugar 0.3 g ;Protein 4.9 g

Jalapeño Poppers

Servings: 12
Cooking Time: 30 Minutes

Ingredients:

- 24 medium jalapeño peppers
- 1 pound uncooked chorizo pork sausage, crumbled
- 2 cups cheddar cheese, shredded
- 12 bacon strips, cut in half

Directions:

1. Cut each jalapeno in half lengthwise, about 1/8-inch deep.
2. Then remove the seeds.
3. In a bowl, place the sausage and cheese and mix well.
4. Stuff the jalapeño peppers with cheese mixture and then wrap each with a piece of bacon.
5. With toothpicks, secure each jalapeño pepper.
6. Place the water tray in the bottom of Hamilton Beach Grill.
7. Place about 2 cups of lukewarm water into the water tray.
8. Place the drip pan over water tray and then, arrange the heating element.
9. Now, place the grilling pan over heating element.
10. Plugin the Hamilton Beach Grill and press the 'Power' button to turn it on.
11. Then press 'Fan" button.
12. Set the temperature settings according to manufacturer's directions.
13. Cover the grill with lid and let it preheat.
14. After preheating, remove the lid and grease the grilling pan.
15. Place the jalapeño peppers over the grilling pan.
16. Cover with the lid and cook for about 35-40 minutes, flipping once halfway through.
17. Discard the toothpicks and serve warm.

Nutrition Info: (Per Serving):Calories 373 ;Total Fat 29.5 g ;Saturated Fat 11.4 g ;Cholesterol 83 mg ;Sodium 1800 mg ;Total Carbs 2.7 g ;Fiber 1.1 g ;Sugar 1 g ;Protein 23.2 g

Zucchini Roulades

Servings: 8
Cooking Time: 12 Minutes

Ingredients:

- 4 medium zucchinis
- 1 cup part-skim ricotta cheese
- ¼ cup Parmesan cheese, grated
- 2 tablespoons fresh basil, minced
- 1 tablespoon Greek olives, chopped
- 1 tablespoon capers, drained
- 1 teaspoon lemon zest, grated
- 1 tablespoon fresh lemon juice
- Salt and ground black pepper, as required

Directions:

1. Cut each zucchini into 1/8-inch thick slices lengthwise.
2. Place the water tray in the bottom of Hamilton Beach Grill.
3. Place about 2 cups of lukewarm water into the water tray.
4. Place the drip pan over water tray and then arrange the heating element.
5. Now, place the grilling pan over heating element.
6. Plugin the Hamilton Beach Grill and press the 'Power' button to turn it on.
7. Then press 'Fan" button.
8. Set the temperature settings according to manufacturer's directions.
9. After preheating, remove the lid and grease the grilling pan.
10. Place half of the zucchini slices over the grilling pan.
11. Cover with the lid and cook for about 2-3 minutes per side.
12. Transfer the zucchini slices onto a platter.
13. Repeat with the remaining slices.
14. Meanwhile, in a small bowl, place the remaining ingredients and mix well. Set aside.
15. Place about 1 tablespoon of cheese mixture on the end of each zucchini slice.
16. Roll up and secure each with a toothpick.
17. Serve immediately.

Nutrition Info: (Per Serving):Calories 70 ;Total Fat 3.4 g ;Saturated Fat 1.9 g ;Cholesterol 12 mg ;Sodium 131 mg ;Total Carbs 5.1 g ;Fiber 1.2 g ;Sugar 1.9 g ;Protein 5.8 g

Veggie Burger

Servings: 5
Cooking Time: 5 Minutes
Ingredients:
- 1 cup cooked brown rice
- 1 cup raw walnuts, finely chopped
- 1/2 tablespoons avocado oil
- 1/2 medium white onion, diced
- 1 tablespoon chili powder
- 1 tablespoon cumin powder
- 1 tablespoon smoked paprika
- 1/2 teaspoons sea salt
- 1/2 teaspoons black pepper
- 1 tablespoon coconut sugar
- 1 ½ cups cooked black beans, drained
- 1/3 cup panko bread crumbs
- 4 tablespoons BBQ sauce

Directions:
1. Add brown rice, walnuts, and all the veggies burger ingredients to a food processor.
2. Blend this mixture for 3 minutes then transfer to a bowl.
3. Make 5 patties out of this vegetable beans mixture.
4. Turn the "Selector" knob to the "Grill Panini" side.
5. Preheat the bottom grill of Hamilton Beach Grill at 350 degrees F and the upper grill plate on medium heat.
6. Once it is preheated, open the lid and place the veggie burgers in the Griddler.
7. Close the griddler's lid and grill the burgers for 5 minutes.
8. Serve warm.

Nutrition Info: (Per Serving): Calories 213 ;Total Fat 14 g ;Saturated Fat 8 g ;Cholesterol 81 mg ;Sodium 162 mg ;Total Carbs 23 g ;Fiber 0.7 g ;Sugar 19 g ;Protein 12 g

Italian-seasoned Grilled Veggies

Servings: 8

Cooking Time: 8 Minutes

Ingredients:

- 1 Zucchini, cut into chunks
- 1 Squash, cut into chunks
- 8 ounces Button Mushrooms, quartered
- 1 Red Bell Pepper, chopped
- 1 Red Onion, cut into chunks
- 2 tbsp Balsamic Vinegar
- 4 tbsp Olive Oil
- 2 tbsp Italian Seasoning
- 4 tbsp grated Parmesan Cheese
- Juice of 1 Lemon
- ½ tsp Garlic Powder

Directions:

1. Preheat your grill to medium-high heat.
2. In a bowl, place all of the ingredient, except the Parmesan Cheese.
3. With your hands, mix well so that each chunk of veggie is coated with oil and seasoning.
4. Thread the veggie chunks onto metal skewers (You can also use soaked wooden ones).
5. When the grill is ready, open the lid, and arrange the skewers onto the bottom plate.
6. Without covering the lid, cook for about 4 minutes.
7. Flip the skewers over and cook for another 3-4 minutes.
8. Serve sprinkled with Parmesan cheese and enjoy!

Nutrition Info: Calories 110 ;Total Fats 8g ;Carbs 7.5g ;Protein 3g ;Fiber: 2.5g

Bacon-wrapped Asparagus

Servings: 4
Cooking Time: 12 Minutes

Ingredients:

- 12 fresh asparagus spears, trimmed
- Olive oil cooking spray
- 1/8 teaspoon ground black pepper
- 6 bacon strips, halved lengthwise

Directions:

1. Spray the asparagus spears wit cooing spry evenly.
2. Wrap a bacon piece around each asparagus spear and then secure ends with toothpicks.
3. Place the water tray in the bottom of Hamilton Beach Grill.
4. Place about 2 cups of lukewarm water into the water tray.
5. Place the drip pan over water tray and then arrange the heating element.
6. Now, place the grilling pan over heating element.
7. Plugin the Hamilton Beach Grill and press the 'Power' button to turn it on.
8. Then press 'Fan" button.
9. Set the temperature settings according to manufacturer's directions.
10. Cover the grill with lid and let it preheat.
11. After preheating, remove the lid and grease the grilling pan.
12. Place the asparagus spears over the grilling pan.
13. Cover with the lid and cook for about 4-6 minutes per side.
14. Discard the toothpicks and serve warm.

Nutrition Info: (Per Serving):Calories 250 ;Total Fat 18.3 g ;Saturated Fat 6 g ;Cholesterol 48 mg ;Sodium 1004 mg ;Total Carbs 3.5 g ;Fiber 1.5 g ;Sugar 1.4 g ;Protein 17.7 g

Charred Tofu

Servings: 3
Cooking Time: 15 Minutes

Ingredients:

- 12 ounces extra-firm tofu, pressed, drained and cut into ½-inch thick slices
- Salt and ground black pepper, as required

Directions:

1. Season the tofu slices with salt and pepper.
2. Place the water tray in the bottom of Hamilton Beach Grill.
3. Place about 2 cups of lukewarm water into the water tray.
4. Place the drip pan over water tray and then arrange the heating element.
5. Now, place the grilling pan over heating element.
6. Plugin the Hamilton Beach Grill and press the 'Power' button to turn it on.
7. Then press 'Fan" button.
8. Set the temperature settings according to manufacturer's directions.
9. Cover the grill with lid and let it preheat.
10. After preheating, remove the lid and grease the grilling pan.
11. Place the mushrooms over the grilling pan.
12. Cover with the lid and cook for about 10-15 minutes, flipping once halfway through.
13. Serve warm.

Nutrition Info: (Per Serving):Calories 103 ;Total Fat 6.6 g ;Saturated Fat 0.6 g ;Cholesterol 0 mg ;Sodium 59 mg ;Total Carbs 2.3 g ;Fiber 0.5 g ;Sugar 0.6 g ;Protein 11.2 g

Grilled Veggies

Servings: 2

Cooking Time: 8 Minutes

Ingredients:

- 1 eggplant, sliced
- 1 zucchini, sliced
- 1 onion, sliced
- 2 tablespoons olive oil
- 1 tablespoon kosher salt
- 1 tablespoon black pepper

Directions:

1. Toss and season all the vegetable slices with oil, black pepper and salt.
2. Turn the "Selector" knob to the "Grill Panini" side.
3. Preheat the bottom grill of Hamilton Beach Grill at 350 degrees F and the upper grill plate on medium heat.
4. Once it is preheated, open the lid and place the vegetables in the Griddler.
5. Close the griddler's lid and grill the veggies for 8 minutes until lightly charred.
6. Serve warm.

Nutrition Info: (Per Serving): Calories 246 ;Total Fat 14.8 g ;Saturated Fat 0.7 g ;Cholesterol 22 mg ;Sodium 220 mg ;Total Carbs 10.3 g ;Fiber 2.4 g ;Sugar 1.2 g ;Protein 12.4 g

Sriracha Wings

Servings: 8
Cooking Time: 18 Minutes
Ingredients:
- For Wings:
- 3 pounds chicken wings
- 1 tablespoon canola oil
- 2 teaspoons ground coriander
- ½ teaspoon garlic salt
- ¼ teaspoon ground black pepper
- For Sauce:
- ½ cup fresh orange juice
- 1/3 cup Sriracha chili sauce
- ¼ cup butter, melted
- 3 tablespoons honey
- 2 tablespoons lime juice
- ¼ cup fresh cilantro, chopped

Directions:
1. For wings: in a bowl, place all ingredients and toss to coat well.
2. Cover the bowl and refrigerate for about 2 hours or overnight.
3. For sauce: in a bowl, place orange juice, chili sauce, butter, honey and lime juice and mix until well combined. Set aside.
4. Place the water tray in the bottom of Hamilton Beach Grill.
5. Place about 2 cups of lukewarm water into the water tray.
6. Place the drip pan over water tray and then, arrange the heating element.
7. Now, place the grilling pan over heating element.
8. Plugin the Hamilton Beach Grill and press the 'Power' button to turn it on.
9. Then press 'Fan" button.
10. Set the temperature settings according to manufacturer's directions.
11. Cover the grill with lid and let it preheat.
12. After preheating, remove the lid and grease the grilling pan.
13. Place the chicken wings over the grilling pan.
14. Cover with the lid and cook for about 15-18 minutes, flipping occasionally.
15. In the last 5 minutes of cooking, brush the wings with some of the sauce.
16. Transfer chicken into the bowl of the remaining sauce and toss to coat.
17. Garnish with cilantro and serve.

Nutrition Info: (Per Serving):Calories 432 ;Total Fat 20.1 g ;Saturated Fat 7.3 g ;Cholesterol 167 mg ;Sodium 258 mg ;Total Carbs 10.5 g ;Fiber 0.1 g ;Sugar 7.9 g ;Protein 49.5 g

Mayo & Parmesan Corn On The Cob

Servings: 4

Cooking Time: 15 Minutes

Ingredients:

- 4 Ears of Corn
- 1 cup grated Parmesan Cheese
- ½ cup Mayonnaise
- Juice of 1 Lemon
- 1 cup Sour Cream
- ½ tsp Cayenne Pepper
- 4 tbsp chopped Cilantro

Directions:

1. Preheat your grill to medium-high heat.
2. Clean the corn by removing the husk and silk.
3. When the grill is ready, open the lid and place the corn on top of the bottom plate.
4. Cook for about 10 to 15 minutes, rotating occasionally while grilling.
5. Meanwhile, combine the sour cream, mayonnaise, and cilantro.
6. Brush the grilled corn with this mixture, and generously sprinkle with Parmesan cheese.
7. Drizzle the lime juice over before serving. Enjoy!

Nutrition Info: Calories 428 ;Total Fats 34g ;Carbs 22g ;Protein 11g ;Fiber: 2g

POULTRY RECIPES

Simple Cajun Chicken Legs

Servings: 1

Cooking Time: 8 Minutes

Ingredients:

- 8 Chicken Legs, boneless
- 2 tbsp Olive Oil
- 2 tbsp Cajun Seasoning

Directions:

1. Preheat your grill to medium-high.
2. Brush them with the olive oil, and then rub the legs with the seasoning.
3. When the green light is on, arrange the legs onto the bottom plate.
4. Lower the lid, and let the legs cook closed, for about 8 to 10 minutes.
5. Serve with the favorite side dish, Enjoy!

Nutrition Info: Calories 370 ;Total Fats 19.2g ;Carbs 0.5g ;Protein 35g ;Fiber: 0g

Spicy Chicken Thighs

Servings: 3
Cooking Time: 18 Minutes

Ingredients:

- 2 tablespoons fresh lime juice
- 1 tablespoon ground chipotle powder
- 1 tablespoon paprika
- 1 tablespoon dried oregano, crushed
- ½ tablespoon garlic powder
- Salt and ground black pepper, as required
- 6 (4-ounce) skinless, boneless chicken thighs

Directions:

1. In a bowl, add all ingredients except chicken thighs and mix until well combined.
2. Coat the thighs with spice mixture generously.
3. Place the water tray in the bottom of Hamilton Beach Grill.
4. Place about 2 cups of lukewarm water into the water tray.
5. Place the drip pan over water tray and then arrange the heating element.
6. Now, place the grilling pan over heating element.
7. Plugin the Hamilton Beach Grill and press the 'Power' button to turn it on.
8. Then press 'Fan" button.
9. Set the temperature settings according to manufacturer's directions.
10. Cover the grill with lid and let it preheat.
11. After preheating, remove the lid and grease the grilling pan.
12. Place the chicken thighs over the grilling pan.
13. Cover with the lid and cook for about 8 minutes.
14. Carefully change the side and grill for 8-10 minutes more.
15. Serve hot.

Nutrition Info: (Per Serving):Calories 300 ;Total Fat 8.6 g ;Saturated Fat 3.1 g ;Cholesterol 132 mg ;Sodium 133 mg ;Total Carbs 3.4 g ;Fiber 1.6 g ;Sugar 0.6 g ;Protein 51.4 g

Glazed Chicken Drumsticks

Servings: 12

Cooking Time: 25 Minutes

Ingredients:

- 1 (10-ounce) jar red jalapeño pepper jelly
- ¼ cup fresh lime juice
- 12 (6-ounce) chicken drumsticks
- Salt and ground black pepper, as required

Directions:

1. In a small saucepan, add jelly and lime juice over medium heat and cook for about 3-5 minutes or until melted.
2. Remove from the heat and set aside.
3. Sprinkle the chicken drumsticks with salt and black pepper.
4. Place the water tray in the bottom of Hamilton Beach Grill.
5. Place about 2 cups of lukewarm water into the water tray.
6. Place the drip pan over water tray and then arrange the heating element.
7. Now, place the grilling pan over heating element.
8. Plugin the Hamilton Beach Grill and press the 'Power' button to turn it on.
9. Then press 'Fan" button.
10. Set the temperature settings according to manufacturer's directions.
11. Cover the grill with lid and let it preheat.
12. After preheating, remove the lid and grease the grilling pan.
13. Place the chicken drumsticks over the grilling pan.
14. Cover with the lid and cook for about 15-20 minutes, flipping occasionally.
15. In the last 5 minutes of cooking, baste the chicken thighs with jelly mixture.
16. Serve hot.

Nutrition Info: (Per Serving):Calories 359 ;Total Fat 9.7 g ;Saturated Fat 2.6 g ;Cholesterol 150 mg ;Sodium 155 mg ;Total Carbs 17.1 g ;Fiber 0 g ;Sugar 11.4 g ;Protein 46.8 g

Marinated Chicken Kabobs

Servings: 4
Cooking Time: 15 Minutes
Ingredients:
- 1/3 cup extra-virgin olive oil, divided
- 2 garlic cloves, minced
- 1 tablespoon fresh rosemary, minced
- 1 tablespoon fresh oregano, minced
- 1 teaspoon fresh lemon zest, grated
- ½ teaspoon red chili flakes, crushed
- 1 pound boneless, skinless chicken breast, cut into ¾-inch cubes
- 1¾ cups green seedless grapes, rinsed
- ½ teaspoon salt
- 1 tablespoon fresh lemon juice

Directions:
1. In small bowl, add ¼ cup of oil, garlic, fresh herbs, lemon zest and chili flakes and beat until well combined.
2. Thread the chicken cubes and grapes onto 12 metal skewers.
3. In a large baking dish, arrange the skewers.
4. Place the marinade and mix well.
5. Refrigerate to marinate for about 4-24 hours.
6. Place the water tray in the bottom of Hamilton Beach Grill.
7. Place about 2 cups of lukewarm water into the water tray.
8. Place the drip pan over water tray and then arrange the heating element.
9. Now, place the grilling pan over heating element.
10. Plugin the Hamilton Beach Grill and press the 'Power' button to turn it on.
11. Then press 'Fan" button.
12. Set the temperature settings according to manufacturer's directions.
13. Cover the grill with lid and let it preheat.
14. After preheating, remove the lid and grease the grilling pan.
15. Place the chicken skewers over the grilling pan.
16. Cover with the lid and cook for about 3-5 minutes per side or until chicken is done completely.
17. Remove from the grill and transfer the skewers onto a serving platter.
18. Drizzle with lemon juice and remaining oil and serve.

Nutrition Info: (Per Serving):Calories 310 ;Total Fat 20.1 g ;Saturated Fat 2.6 g ;Cholesterol 73 mg ;Sodium 351 mg ;Total Carbs 8.8 g ;Fiber 1.3 g ;Sugar 6.7 g ;Protein 24.6 g

Whiskey Wings

Servings: 4

Cooking Time: 6 Minutes

Ingredients:

- 1 tbsp Whiskey
- 1/2 tbsp Chili Powder
- 1 tsp Paprika
- 20 Chicken Wings
- ¼ tsp Garlic Powder
- Salt and Pepper, to taste
- 2 tsp Brown Sugar

Directions:

1. Preheat your grill to 375 degrees F.
2. In the meantime, dump all of the ingredients in a large bowl.
3. With your hands, mix well, to coat the chicken wings completely.
4. When the green light is on, open the grill and arrange the chicken wings onto it.
5. Lower the lid and cook closed for 6 minutes. You can check near the end to see if you need to increase (or decrease) the grilling time for your preferred doneness.
6. Serve with rice and enjoy!

Nutrition Info: Calories 210 ;Total Fats 21g ;Carbs 9.3g ;Protein 18g ;Fiber: 0g

Marinated Chicken Breasts

Servings: 4
Cooking Time: 16 Minutes

Ingredients:

- ¼ cup extra-virgin olive oil
- 2 tablespoons fresh lemon juice
- 2 tablespoons maple syrup
- 1 garlic clove, minced
- Salt and ground black pepper, as required
- 4 (6-ounce) boneless, skinless chicken breasts

Directions:

1. For marinade: in a large bowl, add oil, lemon juice, maple syrup, garlic, salt and black pepper and beat until well combined.
2. In a large resealable plastic bag, place the chicken and marinade.
3. Seal the bag and shake to coat well.
4. Refrigerate overnight.
5. Place the water tray in the bottom of Hamilton Beach Grill.
6. Place about 2 cups of lukewarm water into the water tray.
7. Place the drip pan over water tray and then arrange the heating element.
8. Now, place the grilling pan over heating element.
9. Plugin the Hamilton Beach Grill and press the 'Power' button to turn it on.
10. Then press 'Fan" button.
11. Set the temperature settings according to manufacturer's directions.
12. Cover the grill with lid and let it preheat.
13. After preheating, remove the lid and grease the grilling pan.
14. Place the chicken breasts over the grilling pan.
15. Cover with the lid and cook for about 5-8 minutes per side.
16. Serve hot.

Nutrition Info: (Per Serving):Calories 460 ;Total Fat 25.3 g ;Saturated Fat 5.3 g ;Cholesterol 151 mg ;Sodium 188 mg ;Total Carbs 7.1 g ;Fiber 0.1 g ;Sugar 6.1 g ;Protein 49.3 g

Duck Veggie Kebobs

Servings: 2
Cooking Time: 7 Minutes

Ingredients:

- 8 ounces boneless and skinless Duck (breast is fine)
- 1/2 small Squash
- ½ Zucchini
- 1 small Red Bell Pepper
- ¼ Red Onion
- 2 tbsp Olive Oil
- 1 tbsp Balsamic Vinegar
- 2 tsp Dijon Mustard
- 2 tsp Honey
- Salt and Pepper, to taste

Directions:

1. Whisk together the oil, vinegar, mustard, honey, and some salt and pepper, in a bowl.
2. Cut the duck into chunks and dump into the bowl.
3. Mix to coat well and set aside. You can leave in the fridge for an hour or two, but if you are in a hurry, you can place on the grill straight away – it will taste great, as well.
4. Cut the veggies into chunks.
5. Plug the grill in, and set the temperature to 375 degrees F.
6. Thread the duck and veggies onto metallic skewers.
7. Open the grill and place on the bottom plate.
8. Lower the lid and cook for 5-8 minutes, depending on how done you want the meat to be.
9. Serve and enjoy!

Nutrition Info: Calories 250 ;Total Fats 10g ;Carbs 11g ;Protein 30g ;Fiber: 2g

Basil Grilled Chicken With Asparagus

Servings: 4

Cooking Time: 7 Minutes

Ingredients:

- 1 tsp Dijon Mustard
- 1 pound boneless and skinless Chicken Breasts
- 1 tsp dried Basil
- 1 tsp minced Garlic
- 2 tbsp Olive Oil
- ¼ tsp Onion Powder
- 12 Asparagus Spears
- Salt and Pepper, to taste

Directions:

1. Combine the oil, mustard, basil, garlic, onion powder, and some salt and pepper, in a bowl.
2. Coat the chicken with this mixture.
3. Meanwhile, preheat your grill to 350 degrees F.
4. Arrange the chicken breasts onto the bottom plate.
5. Season the asparagus with salt and pepper and add them next to the chicken.
6. Lower the lid, and cook closed, for 7 full minutes, or until your preferred doneness is reached.
7. Serve and enjoy!

Nutrition Info: Calories 350 ;Total Fats 24g ;Carbs 6g ;Protein 26g ;Fiber: 2g

Tequila Chicken

Servings: 3
Cooking Time: 7 Minutes

Ingredients:

- 1/2 cup gold tequila
- 1 cup lime juice
- 1/2 cup orange juice
- 1 tablespoon chili powder
- 1 tablespoon minced jalapeno pepper
- 1 tablespoon minced fresh garlic
- 2 teaspoons kosher salt
- 1 teaspoon black pepper
- 3 boneless chicken breasts

Directions:

1. Mix tequila, lime juice, orange juice, chili powder, jalapeno pepper, garlic, black pepper and salt in a bowl.
2. Add chicken breasts to the tequila marinade, cover and marinate for 1 hour.
3. Turn the "Selector" knob to the "Grill Panini" side.
4. Preheat the bottom grill of Hamilton Beach Grill at 350 degrees F and the upper grill plate on medium heat.
5. Once it is preheated, open the lid and place the chicken breasts in the Griddler.
6. Close the griddler's lid and grill the chicken breasts for 7 minutes.
7. Serve warm.

Nutrition Info: (Per Serving): Calories 352 ;Total Fat 14 g ;Saturated Fat 2 g ;Cholesterol 65 mg ;Sodium 220 mg ;Total Carbs 15.8 g ;Fiber 0.2 g ;Sugar 1 g ;Protein 26 g

Meatballs Kabobs

Servings: 4
Cooking Time: 14 Minutes
Ingredients:
- 1 yellow onion, chopped roughly
- ½ cup lemongrass, chopped roughly
- 2 garlic cloves, chopped roughly
- 1½ pounds lean ground turkey
- 1 teaspoon sesame oil
- ½ tablespoons low-sodium soy sauce
- 1 tablespoon arrowroot starch
- 1/8 teaspoons powdered stevia
- Salt and ground black pepper, as required

Directions:
1. In a food processor, add the onion, lemongrass and garlic and pulse until chopped finely.
2. Transfer the onion mixture into a large bowl.
3. Add the remaining ingredients and mix until well combined.
4. Make 12 equal sized balls from meat mixture.
5. Thread the balls onto the presoaked wooden skewers.
6. Place the water tray in the bottom of Hamilton Beach Grill.
7. Place about 2 cups of lukewarm water into the water tray.
8. Place the drip pan over water tray and then arrange the heating element.
9. Now, place the grilling pan over heating element.
10. Plugin the Hamilton Beach Grill and press the 'Power' button to turn it on.
11. Then press 'Fan" button.
12. Set the temperature settings according to manufacturer's directions.
13. Cover the grill with lid and let it preheat.
14. After preheating, remove the lid and grease the grilling pan.
15. Place the skewers over the grilling pan.
16. Cover with the lid and cook for about 6-7 minutes per side.
17. Serve hot.

Nutrition Info: (Per Serving):Calories 276 ;Total Fat 13.4 g ;Saturated Fat 4 g ;Cholesterol 122 mg ;Sodium 280 mg ;Total Carbs 5.6 g ;Fiber 0.6 g ;Sugar 1.3 g ;Protein 34.2 g

Ketchup Glaze Chicken Thighs

Servings: 12

Cooking Time: 16 Minutes

Ingredients:

- ½ cup packed brown sugar
- 1/3 cup ketchup
- 1/3 cup low-sodium soy sauce
- 3 tablespoons sherry
- 1½ teaspoons fresh ginger root, minced
- 1½ teaspoons garlic, minced
- 12 (6-ounce) boneless, skinless chicken thighs

Directions:

1. In a small bowl, place all ingredients except for chicken thighs and mix well.
2. Transfer about 1 1/3 cups for marinade in another bowl and refrigerate.
3. In a zip lock bag, add the remaining marinade and chicken thighs.
4. Seal the bag and shake to coat well.
5. Refrigerate overnight.
6. Remove the chicken thighs from bag and discard the marinade.
7. Place the water tray in the bottom of Hamilton Beach Grill.
8. Place about 2 cups of lukewarm water into the water tray.
9. Place the drip pan over water tray and then arrange the heating element.
10. Now, place the grilling pan over heating element.
11. Plugin the Hamilton Beach Grill and press the 'Power' button to turn it on.
12. Then press 'Fan" button.
13. Set the temperature settings according to manufacturer's directions.
14. Cover the grill with lid and let it preheat.
15. After preheating, remove the lid and grease the grilling pan.
16. Place the chicken thighs over the grilling pan.
17. Cover with the lid and cook for about 6-8 minutes per side.
18. In the last 5 minutes of cooking, baste the chicken thighs with reserved marinade.
19. Serve hot.

Nutrition Info: (Per Serving):Calories 359 ;Total Fat 12.6 g ;Saturated Fat 3.6 g ;Cholesterol 151 mg ;Sodium 614 mg ;Total Carbs 8.3 g ;Fiber 0 g ;Sugar 7.6 g ;Protein 49.8 g

Lemon And Rosemary Turkey And Zucchini Threads

Servings: 4

Cooking Time: 7 Minutes

Ingredients:

- 1-pound Turkey Breasts, boneless and skinless
- 1 Large Zuchinni
- 2 tbsp Lemon Juice
- ½ tsp Lemon Zest
- ¼ cup Olive Oil
- 1 tbsp Honey
- 1 tbsp Fresh Rosemary
- ¼ tsp Garlic Powder
- Salt and Pepper, to taste

Directions:

1. Cut the Turkey into smaller chunks, and place inside a bowl.
2. Add the olive oil, lemon juice, zest, honey, rosemary, garlic powder, and some salt and pepper, to the bowl.
3. With your hands, mix well until the turkey is completely coated with the mixture.
4. Cover and let sit in the fridge for about an hour.
5. Wash the zucchini thoroughly and cut into small chunks. Season with salt and pepper.
6. Preheat your Grill to 350 – 375 degrees F.
7. Thread the turkey and zucchini onto soaked (or metal) skewers and arrange on the bottom plate.
8. Lower the lid and cook closed for 6-7 minutes.
9. Serve and enjoy!

Nutrition Info: Calories 280 ;Total Fats 23g ;Carbs 6g ;Protein 27g ;Fiber: 0.5g

Grilled Chicken Skewers

Servings: 4

Cooking Time: 5 Minutes

Ingredients:

- 1/4 cup fresh lime juice
- 2 garlic cloves, sliced
- 1 chipotle chile in adobo, chopped
- Kosher salt and black pepper, to taste
- 2 boneless chicken breasts, cut into chunks

Directions:

1. Mix chicken cubes with black pepper, salt, chile, garlic and lime juice in a bowl.
2. Thread the chicken cubes on the wooden skewers.
3. Turn the "Selector" knob to the "Grill Panini" side.
4. Preheat the bottom grill of Hamilton Beach Grill at 350 degrees F and the upper grill plate on medium heat.
5. Once it is preheated, open the lid and place the skewers in the Griddler.
6. Close the griddler's lid and grill the skewers for 5 minutes.
7. Serve warm.

Nutrition Info: (Per Serving): Calories 440 ;Total Fat 7.9 g ;Saturated Fat 1.8 g ;Cholesterol 5 mg ;Sodium 581 mg ;Total Carbs 21.8 g ;Sugar 7.1 g ;Fiber 2.6 g ;Protein 37.2 g

Grilled Chicken Breast

Servings: 2

Cooking Time: 12 Minutes

Ingredients:

- 3 tablespoons olive oil
- 5 fresh basil leaves, torn
- 1 clove garlic, sliced
- 2 chicken breasts, boneless, skinless
- Kosher salt and black pepper, to taste

Directions:

1. Rub the chicken breasts with black pepper, salt, garlic, basil leaves and olive oil.
2. Turn the "Selector" knob to the "Grill Panini" side.
3. Preheat the bottom grill of Hamilton Beach Grill at 350 degrees F and the upper grill plate on medium heat.
4. Once it is preheated, open the lid and place the chicken breasts in the Griddler.
5. Close the griddler's lid and grill the skewers for 12 minutes.
6. Serve warm.

Nutrition Info: (Per Serving): Calories 453 ;Total Fat 2.4 g ;Saturated Fat 3 g ;Cholesterol 21 mg ;Sodium 216 mg ;Total Carbs 18 g ;Fiber 2.3 g ;Sugar 1.2 g ;Protein 23.2 g

Grilled Duck Breasts

Servings: 4
Cooking Time: 6 Minutes
Ingredients:

- 1/4 cup olive oil
- 1 tablespoon dried oregano
- 2 pounds duck breasts
- 3 large garlic cloves, grated
- 2 lemons
- Kosher salt and black pepper, to taste

Directions:

1. Rub the duck breast with black pepper, salt, lemon juice, garlic, oregano and olive oil.
2. Place the duck breasts in a plate, cover and marinate for 30 minutes.
3. Turn the "Selector" knob to the "Grill Panini" side.
4. Preheat the bottom grill of Hamilton Beach Grill at 350 degrees F and the upper grill plate on medium heat.
5. Once it is preheated, open the lid and place the duck breasts in the Griddler.
6. Close the griddler's lid and grill the duck for 6 minutes.
7. Serve warm.

Nutrition Info: (Per Serving): Calories 301 ;Total Fat 15.8 g ;Saturated Fat 2.7 g ;Cholesterol 75 mg ;Sodium 189 mg ;Total Carbs 31.7 g ;Fiber 0.3 g ;Sugar 0.1 g ;Protein 28.2 g

Lemon Grilled Chicken Thighs

Servings: 4

Cooking Time: 6 Minutes

Ingredients:

- Juice and zest of 2 lemons
- 2 sprigs fresh rosemary, chopped
- 2 sprigs fresh sage, chopped
- 2 garlic cloves, smashed and chopped
- 1/4 teaspoon crushed red pepper
- 4 chicken thighs, trimmed
- Kosher salt, to taste

Directions:

1. Rub the chicken thighs with salt, oil, red pepper, garlic, sage, rosemary, lemon zest and juice.
2. Place the chicken in a bowl, cover and marinate for 1 hour for marination.
3. Turn the "Selector" knob to the "Grill Panini" side.
4. Preheat the bottom grill of Hamilton Beach Grill at 350 degrees F and the upper grill plate on medium heat.
5. Once it is preheated, open the lid and place 2 chicken thighs in the Griddler.
6. Close the griddler's lid and grill the chicken for 6 minutes.
7. Transfer them to a plate and grill the remaining thighs.
8. Serve warm.

Nutrition Info: (Per Serving): Calories 388 ;Total Fat 8 g ;Saturated Fat 1 g ;Cholesterol 153mg ;sodium 339 mg ;Total Carbs 8 g ;Fiber 1 g ;Sugar 2 g ;Protein 13 g

Teriyaki Chicken Thighs

Servings: 4

Cooking Time: 7 Minutes

Ingredients:

- 4 Chicken Thighs
- ½ cup Brown Sugar
- ½ cup Teriyaki Sauce
- 2 tbsp Rice Vinegar
- 1 thumb-sized piece of Ginger, minced
- ¼ cup Water
- 2 tsp minced Garlic
- 1 tbsp Cornstarch

Directions:

1. Place the sugar, teriyaki sauce, vinegar, ginger, water, and garlic, in a bowl.
2. Mix to combine well.
3. Transfer half of the mixture to a saucepan and set aside.
4. Add the chicken thighs to the bowl, and coat well.
5. Cover the bowl with wrap, and place in the fridge. Let sit for one hour.
6. Preheat your grill to medium.
7. In the meantime, place the saucepan over medium heat and add the cornstarch. Cook until thickened. Remove from heat and set aside.
8. Arrange the thighs onto the preheated bottom and close the lid.
9. Cook for 5 minutes, then open, brush the thickened sauce over, and cover again.
10. Cook for additional minute or two.
11. Serve and enjoy!

Nutrition Info: Calories 321 ;Total Fats 11g ;Carbs 28g ;Protein 31g ;Fiber: 1g

Grilled Honey Chicken

Servings: 4

Cooking Time: 6 Minutes

Ingredients:

- Juice of 2 lemons
- ½ tablespoon Dijon mustard
- 1 tablespoon honey
- A dash of salt
- 2 whole chicken breasts

Directions:

1. Rub the chicken with honey, salt, Dijon and lemon juice.
2. Turn the "Selector" knob to the "Grill Panini" side.
3. Preheat the bottom grill of Hamilton Beach Grill at 350 degrees F and the upper grill plate on medium heat.
4. Once it is preheated, open the lid and place the chicken breasts in the Griddler.
5. Close the griddler's lid and grill the chicken for 6 minutes.
6. Serve warm.

Nutrition Info: (Per Serving): Calories 231 ;Total Fat 20.1 g ;Saturated Fat 2.4 g ;Cholesterol 110 mg ;Sodium 941 mg ;Total Carbs 30.1 g ;Fiber 0.9 g ;Sugar 1.4 g ;Protein 14.6 g

Chicken Yakitori

Servings: 4

Cooking Time: 6 Minutes

Ingredients:

- 2 tbsp Honey
- 1 tsp minced Garlic
- 1-pound boneless Chicken
- 1 tsp minced Ginger
- 4 tbsp Soy Sauce
- Salt and Pepper, to taste

Directions:

1. In a bowl, combine the honey, ginger, soy sauce, and garlic. Add some salt and pepper.
2. Cut the chicken into thick stripes and add them to the bowl.
3. Mix until the meat is completely coated with the marinade.
4. Cover the bowl and refrigerate for about one hour.
5. Preheat your grill to medium.
6. Thread the chicken onto metal (or soaked wooden) skewers and arrange onto the bottom plate.
7. Lower the lid and cook for about 6-7 minutes, depending on how well-cooked you prefer the meat to be.
8. Serve and enjoy!

Nutrition Info: Calories 182 ;Total Fats 9g ;Carbs 10g ;Protein 27g ;Fiber: 0.2g

Chicken Drumsticks

Servings: 5
Cooking Time: 40 Minutes
Ingredients:

- 2 tablespoons avocado oil
- 1 tablespoon fresh lime juice
- 1 teaspoon red chili powder
- 1 teaspoon garlic powder
- Salt, as required
- 5 (8-ounce) chicken drumsticks

Directions:

1. In a mixing bowl, mix avocado oil, lime juice, chili powder and garlic powder and mix well.
2. Add the chicken drumsticks and coat with the marinade generously.
3. Cover the bowl and refrigerate to marinate for about 30-60 minutes.
4. Place the water tray in the bottom of Hamilton Beach Grill.
5. Place about 2 cups of lukewarm water into the water tray.
6. Place the drip pan over water tray and then arrange the heating element.
7. Now, place the grilling pan over heating element.
8. Plugin the Hamilton Beach Grill and press the 'Power' button to turn it on.
9. Then press 'Fan" button.
10. Set the temperature settings according to manufacturer's directions.
11. Cover the grill with lid and let it preheat.
12. After preheating, remove the lid and grease the grilling pan.
13. Place the chicken drumsticks over the grilling pan.
14. Cover with the lid and cook for about 30-40 minutes, flipping after every 5 minutes.
15. Serve hot.

Nutrition Info: (Per Serving):Calories 395 ;Total Fat 13.8 g ;Saturated Fat 3.6 g ;Cholesterol 200 mg ;Sodium 218 mg ;Total Carbs 1 g ;Fiber 0.5 g ;Sugar 0.2 g ;Protein 62.6 g

FISH & SEAFOOD RECIPES

Grilled Scallops

Servings: 4
Cooking Time: 6 Minutes
Ingredients:

- 1-pound Jumbo Scallops
- 1 ½ tbsp Olive Oil
- ½ tsp Garlic Powder
- Salt and Pepper, to taste
- Dressing:
- 1 tbsp chopped Parsley
- 3 tbsp Lemon Juice
- ½ tsp Lemon Zest
- 2 tbsp Olive Oil
- Salt and Pepper, to taste

Directions:

1. Preheat your grill to medium-high.
2. Brush the scallops with olive oi, and sprinkle with salt, pepper, and garlic powder.
3. Arrange onto the bottom plate and cook for about 3 minutes, with the lid off.
4. Flip over, and grill for an additional two or three minutes.
5. Meanwhile, make the dressing by combining all of the ingredients in a small bowl.
6. Transfer the grilled scallops to a serving plate and drizzle the dressing over.
7. Enjoy!

Nutrition Info: Calories 102 ;Total Fats 5g ;Carbs 3g ;Protein 9.5g ;Fiber: 1g

The Easiest Pesto Shrimp

Servings: 2

Cooking Time: 5 Minutes

Ingredients:

- 1-pound Shrimp, tails and shells discarded
- ½ cup Pesto Sauce

Directions:

1. Place the cleaned shrimp in a bowl and add the pesto sauce to it.
2. Mix gently with your hands, until each shrimp is coated with the sauce. Let sit for about 15 minutes.
3. In the meantime, preheat your grill to 350 degrees F.
4. Open the grill and arrange the shrimp onto the bottom plate.
5. Cook with the lid off for about 2-3 minutes. Flip over and cook for an additional 2 minutes.
6. Serve as desired and enjoy!

Nutrition Info: Calories 470 ;Total Fats 28.5g ;Carbs 3g ;Protein 50g ;Fiber: 0g

Herbed Salmon

Servings: 4
Cooking Time: 8 Minutes

Ingredients:

- 2 garlic cloves, minced
- 1 teaspoon dried oregano, crushed
- 1 teaspoon dried basil, crushed
- Salt and ground black pepper, as required
- ¼ cup olive oil
- 2 tablespoons fresh lemon juice
- 4 (4-ounce) salmon fillets

Directions:

1. In a large bowl, add all ingredients except for salmon and mix well.
2. Add the salmon and coat with marinade generously.
3. Cover and refrigerate to marinate for at least 1 hour.
4. Place the water tray in the bottom of Hamilton Beach Grill.
5. Place about 2 cups of lukewarm water into the water tray.
6. Place the drip pan over water tray and then arrange the heating element.
7. Now, place the grilling pan over heating element.
8. Plugin the Hamilton Beach Grill and press the 'Power' button to turn it on.
9. Then press 'Fan" button.
10. Set the temperature settings according to manufacturer's directions.
11. Cover the grill with lid and let it preheat.
12. After preheating, remove the lid and grease the grilling pan.
13. Place the salmon fillets over the grilling pan.
14. Cover with the lid and cook for about 4 minutes per side.
15. Serve hot.

Nutrition Info: (Per Serving):Calories 263 ;Total Fat 19.7 g ;Saturated Fat 2.9 g ;Cholesterol 50 mg ;Sodium 91 mg ;Total Carbs 0.9 g ;Fiber 0.2 g ;Sugar 0.2 g ;Protein 22.2 g

Lemony Salmon

Servings: 4

Cooking Time: 14 Minutes

Ingredients:

- 2 garlic cloves, minced
- 1 tablespoon fresh lemon zest, grated
- 2 tablespoons butter, melted
- 2 tablespoons fresh lemon juice
- Salt and ground black pepper, as required
- 4 (6-ounce) boneless, skinless salmon fillets

Directions:

1. In a bowl, place all ingredients (except salmon fillets) and mix well.
2. Add the salmon fillets and coat with garlic mixture generously.
3. Place the water tray in the bottom of Hamilton Beach Grill.
4. Place about 2 cups of lukewarm water into the water tray.
5. Place the drip pan over water tray and then arrange the heating element.
6. Now, place the grilling pan over heating element.
7. Plugin the Hamilton Beach Grill and press the 'Power' button to turn it on.
8. Then press 'Fan" button.
9. Set the temperature settings according to manufacturer's directions.
10. Cover the grill with lid and let it preheat.
11. After preheating, remove the lid and grease the grilling pan.
12. Place the salmon fillets over the grilling pan.
13. Cover with the lid and cook for about 6-7 minutes per side.
14. Serve immediately.

Nutrition Info: (Per Serving):Calories 281 ;Total Fat 16.3 g ;Saturated Fat 5.2 g ;Cholesterol 90 mg ;Sodium 157 mg ;Total Carbs 1 g ;Fiber 0.2 g ;Sugar 0.3 g ;Protein 33.3 g

Barbecue Squid

Servings: 4
Cooking Time: 3 Minutes

Ingredients:

- 1 ½ pounds skinless squid tubes, sliced
- ⅓ cup red bell pepper, chopped
- 13 fresh red Thai chiles, stemmed
- 6 garlic cloves, minced
- 3 shallots, chopped
- 1 (1-inch) piece fresh ginger, chopped
- 6 tablespoons sugar
- 2 tablespoons soy sauce
- 1 ½ teaspoons black pepper
- ¼ teaspoon salt

Directions:

1. Blend bell pepper, red chilies, shallots, sugar, soy sauce, black pepper and salt in a blender.
2. Transfer this marinade to a Ziplock bag and ad squid tubes.
3. Seal the bag and refrigerate for 1 hour for marination.
4. Turn the "Selector" knob to the "Grill Panini" side.
5. Preheat the bottom grill of Hamilton Beach Grill at 350 degrees F and the upper grill plate on medium heat.
6. Once it is preheated, open the lid and place the squid chunks in the Griddler.
7. Close the griddler's lid and grill the squid for 2-3 minutes.
8. Serve warm.

Nutrition Info: (Per Serving): Calories 248 ;Total Fat 15.7 g ;Saturated Fat 2.7 g ;Cholesterol 75 mg ;Sodium 94 mg ;Total Carbs 31.4 g ;Fiber 0.4 g ;Sugar 3.1 g ;Protein 24.9 g

Ginger Salmon

Servings: 3
Cooking Time: 8 Minutes
Ingredients:
- Sauce:
- ¼ tablespoons rice vinegar
- 1 teaspoons sugar
- 1/8 teaspoon salt
- ¼ tablespoon lime zest, grated
- 1/8 cup lime juice
- ½ tablespoon olive oil
- 1/8 teaspoon ground coriander
- 1/8 teaspoon ground black pepper
- 1/8 cup cilantro, chopped
- ¼ tablespoon onion, chopped
- ½ teaspoon ginger root, minced
- 1 garlic clove, minced
- 1 small cucumber, peeled, chopped
- Salmon:
- 2 tablespoons gingerroot, minced
- ¼ tablespoon lime juice
- ¼ tablespoon olive oil
- Salt, to taste
- Black pepper, to taste
- 3 (6 oz.) salmon fillets

Directions:
1. Start by blending the cucumber with all the sauce ingredients in a blender until smooth.
2. Season and rub the salmon fillets with ginger, oil, salt, black pepper, lime juice.
3. Turn the "Selector" knob to the "Grill Panini" side.
4. Preheat the bottom grill of Hamilton Beach Grill at 350 degrees F and the upper grill plate on medium heat.
5. Once it is preheated, open the lid and place the salmon fillets in the Griddler.
6. Close the griddler's lid and grill the salmon fillets for 8 minutes.
7. Serve warm with cucumber sauce.

Nutrition Info: (Per Serving): Calories 457 ;Total Fat 19.1 g ;Saturated Fat 11 g ;Cholesterol 262 mg ;Sodium 557 mg ;Total Carbs 18.9 g ;Sugar 1.2 g ;Fiber 1.7 g ;Protein 32.5 g

Lime Sea Bass

Servings: 4
Cooking Time: 9 Minutes

Ingredients:

- ½ tsp Garlic Powder
- 4 tbsp Lime Juice
- 4 Sea Bass Fillets
- Salt and Pepper, to taste

Directions:

1. Preheat your grill to 375 degrees F.
2. Brush the fillets with lime juice and sprinkle with garlic powder, salt, and pepper.
3. When the green light is on, open the grill, coat with cooking spray, and arrange the fillets on top.
4. Cook open for 4 minutes. Then flip over and cook for 4-5 more minutes on the other side.
5. Serve with rice or favorite side dish, ad enjoy!

Nutrition Info: Calories 130 ;Total Fats 2.6g ;Carbs 0g ;Protein 24g ;Fiber: 0g

Orange-glazed Salmon

Servings: 4
Cooking Time: 8 Minutes
Ingredients:

- 4 Salmon Fillets
- ½ tsp Garlic Powder
- 1 tsp Paprika
- ¼ tsp Cayenne Pepper
- 1 ¾ tsp Salt
- 1 tbsp Brown Sugar
- ¼ tsp Black Pepper
- Glaze:
- 1 tsp Salt
- 2 tbsp Soy Sauce
- Juice of 1 Orange
- 4 tbsp Maple Syrup

Directions:

1. Preheat your grill to medium and coat with cooking spray.
2. In a small bowl, combine the spices together, and then massage the mixture into the fish.
3. Arrange the salmon onto the bottom plate and cook with the lid off.
4. In the meantime, place the glaze ingredients in a saucepan over medium heat.
5. Cook for a couple of minutes, until thickened.
6. Once the salmon has been cooking for 3 minutes, flip it over.
7. Cook for another 3 minutes.
8. Then, brush with the glaze, lower the lid, and cook for an additional minute.
9. Serve with preferred side dish. Enjoy!

Nutrition Info: Calories 250 ;Total Fats 19g ;Carbs 7g ;Protein 22g ;Fiber: 0g

Blackened Salmon

Servings: 2
Cooking Time: 6 Minutes
Ingredients:
- 1 lb. salmon fillets
- 3 tablespoons butter, melted
- 1 tablespoon lemon pepper
- 1 teaspoon seasoned salt
- 1½ tablespoon smoked paprika
- 1 teaspoon cayenne pepper
- ¾ teaspoon onion salt
- ½ teaspoon dry basil
- ½ teaspoon ground white pepper
- ½ teaspoon ground black pepper
- ¼ teaspoon dry oregano
- ¼ teaspoon ancho chili powder

Directions:
1. Liberally season the salmon fillets with butter and other ingredients.
2. Turn the "Selector" knob to the "Grill Panini" side.
3. Preheat the bottom grill of Hamilton Beach Grill at 350 degrees F and the upper grill plate on medium heat.
4. Once it is preheated, open the lid and place the salmon fillets in the Griddler.
5. Close the griddler's lid and grill the fish fillets for 6 minutes.
6. Serve warm.

Nutrition Info: (Per Serving): Calories 378 ;Total Fat 7 g ;Saturated Fat 8.1 g ;Cholesterol 230 mg ;Sodium 316 mg ;Total Carbs 16.2 g ;Sugar 0.2 g ;Fiber 0.3 g ;Protein 26 g

Buttered Halibut

Servings: 2

Cooking Time: 8 Minutes

Ingredients:

- 2 (4-ounce) haddock fillets
- Salt and ground black pepper, as required
- 1 tablespoon butter, melted

Directions:

1. Sprinkle the fish fillets with salt and black pepper generously.
2. Place the water tray in the bottom of Hamilton Beach Grill.
3. Place about 2 cups of lukewarm water into the water tray.
4. Place the drip pan over water tray and then arrange the heating element.
5. Now, place the grilling pan over heating element.
6. Plugin the Hamilton Beach Grill and press the 'Power' button to turn it on.
7. Then press 'Fan" button.
8. Set the temperature settings according to manufacturer's directions.
9. Cover the grill with lid and let it preheat.
10. After preheating, remove the lid and grease the grilling pan.
11. Place the fish fillets over the grilling pan.
12. Cover with the lid and cook for about 3-4 minutes per side.
13. Remove from the grill and place the haddock fillets onto serving plates.
14. Drizzle with melted butter and serve.

Nutrition Info: (Per Serving):Calories 178 ;Total Fat 6.8 g ;Saturated Fat 3.8 g ;Cholesterol 99 mg ;Sodium 217 mg ;Total Carbs 0 g ;Fiber 0 g ;Sugar 0 g ;Protein 27.6 g

Seasoned Tuna

Servings: 2

Cooking Time: 6 Minutes

Ingredients:

- 2 (6-ounce) yellowfin tuna steaks
- 2 tablespoons blackening seasoning
- Olive oil cooking spray

Directions:

1. Coat the tuna steaks with the blackening seasoning evenly.
2. Then spray tuna steaks with cooking spray.
3. Place the water tray in the bottom of Hamilton Beach Grill.
4. Place about 2 cups of lukewarm water into the water tray.
5. Place the drip pan over water tray and then arrange the heating element.
6. Now, place the grilling pan over heating element.
7. Plugin the Hamilton Beach Grill and press the 'Power' button to turn it on.
8. Then press 'Fan" button.
9. Set the temperature settings according to manufacturer's directions.
10. Cover the grill with lid and let it preheat.
11. After preheating, remove the lid and grease the grilling pan.
12. Place the tuna steaks over the grilling pan.
13. Cover with the lid and cook for about 2-3 minutes per side.
14. Serve hot.

Nutrition Info: (Per Serving):Calories 313 ;Total Fat 10.7 g ;Saturated Fat 2.2 g ;Cholesterol 83 mg ;Sodium 169 mg ;Total Carbs 0 g ;Fiber 0 g ;Sugar 0 g ;Protein 50.9 g

Lemon Pepper Salmon With Cherry Tomatoes And Asparagus

Servings: 4

Cooking Time: 5 Minutes

Ingredients:

- 4 Salmon Fillets
- 8 Cherry Tomatoes
- 12 Asparagus Spears
- 2 tbsp Olive Oil
- ½ tsp Garlic Powder
- 1 tsp Lemon Pepper
- ½ tsp Onion Powder
- Salt, to taste

Directions:

1. Preheat your grill to 375 degrees F and cut the tomatoes in half.
2. Brush the salmon, tomatoes, and sparagus with olive oil, and then sprinkle with the spices.
3. Arrange the salmon fillets, cherry tomatoes, and asparagus spears, onto the bottom plate.
4. Gently, lower the lid, and cook the fish and veggies for about 5-6 minutes, or until you reach your desired doneness (check at the 5th minute).
5. Serve and enjoy!

Nutrition Info: Calories 240 ;Total Fats 14g ;Carbs 3.5g ;Protein 24g ;Fiber: 1.4g

Simple Mahi-mahi

Servings: 4
Cooking Time: 10 Minutes

Ingredients:

- 4 (6-ounce) mahi-mahi fillets
- 2 tablespoons olive oil
- Salt and ground black pepper, as required

Directions:

1. Coat fish fillets with olive oil and season with salt and black pepper evenly.
2. Place the water tray in the bottom of Hamilton Beach Grill.
3. Place about 2 cups of lukewarm water into the water tray.
4. Place the drip pan over water tray and then arrange the heating element.
5. Now, place the grilling pan over heating element.
6. Plugin the Hamilton Beach Grill and press the 'Power' button to turn it on.
7. Then press 'Fan" button.
8. Set the temperature settings according to manufacturer's directions.
9. Cover the grill with lid and let it preheat.
10. After preheating, remove the lid and grease the grilling pan.
11. Place the fish fillets over the grilling pan.
12. Cover with the lid and cook for about 5 minutes per side.
13. Serve hot.

Nutrition Info: (Per Serving):Calories 195 ;Total Fat 7 g ;Saturated Fat 1 g ;Cholesterol 60 mg ;Sodium 182 mg ;Total Carbs 0 g ;Fiber 0 g ;Sugar 0 g ;Protein 31.6 g

Salmon Lime Burgers

Servings: 2

Cooking Time: 6 Minutes

Ingredients:

- 1-lb. skinless salmon fillets, minced
- 2 tablespoons grated lime zest
- 1 tablespoon Dijon mustard
- 3 tablespoons shallot, chopped
- 2 tablespoons fresh cilantro, minced
- 1 tablespoon soy sauce
- 1 tablespoon honey
- 3 garlic cloves, minced
- 1/2 teaspoon salt
- 1/4 teaspoon black pepper

Directions:

1. Thoroughly mix all the ingredients for burgers in a bowl.
2. Make four patties out this salmon mixture.
3. Turn the "Selector" knob to the "Grill Panini" side.
4. Preheat the bottom grill of Hamilton Beach Grill at 350 degrees F and the upper grill plate on medium heat.
5. Once it is preheated, open the lid and place the salmon burgers in the Griddler.
6. Close the griddler's lid and grill the salmon burgers for 6 minutes.
7. Serve warm with buns.

Nutrition Info: (Per Serving): Calories 408 ;Total Fat 21 g ;Saturated Fat 4.3 g ;Cholesterol 150 mg ;Sodium 146 mg ;Total Carbs 21.1 g ;Sugar 0.1 g ;Fiber 0.4 g ;Protein 23 g

Shrimp Kabobs

Servings: 6
Cooking Time: 8 Minutes
Ingredients:

- 1 jalapeño pepper, chopped
- 1 large garlic clove, chopped
- 1 (1-inch) fresh ginger, mined
- 1/3 cup fresh mint leaves
- 1 cup coconut milk
- ¼ cup fresh lime juice
- 1 tablespoon red boat fish sauce
- 24 medium shrimp, peeled and deveined
- 1 avocado, peeled, pitted and cubed
- 3 cups seedless watermelon, cubed

Directions:

1. In a food processor, add jalapeño, garlic, ginger, mint, coconut milk, lime juice and fish sauce and pulse until smooth.
2. Add shrimp and coat with marinade generously.
3. Cover and refrigerate to marinate for at least 1-2 hours.
4. Remove shrimp from marinade and thread onto pre-soaked wooden skewers with avocado and watermelon.
5. Place the water tray in the bottom of Hamilton Beach Grill.
6. Place about 2 cups of lukewarm water into the water tray.
7. Place the drip pan over water tray and then arrange the heating element.
8. Now, place the grilling pan over heating element.
9. Plugin the Hamilton Beach Grill and press the 'Power' button to turn it on.
10. Then press 'Fan" button.
11. Set the temperature settings according to manufacturer's directions.
12. Cover the grill with lid and let it preheat.
13. After preheating, remove the lid and grease the grilling pan.
14. Place the skewers over the grilling pan.
15. Cover with the lid and cook for about 3-4 minutes per side.
16. Serve hot.

Nutrition Info: (Per Serving):Calories 294 ;Total Fat 17.7 g ;Saturated Fat 10.4 g ;Cholesterol 185mg ;Sodium 473 mg ;Total Carbs 12.9 g ;Fiber 3.8 g ;Sugar 6.2 g ;Protein 22.9 g;

Tuna Steak With Avocado & Mango Salsa

Servings: 2

Cooking Time: 8 Minutes

Ingredients:

- 2 Tuna Steaks
- 1 ½ tbsp Olive Oil
- 1 tsp Paprika
- 2 tbsp Coconut Sugar
- 1 tsp Onion Powder
- ¼ tsp Pepper
- ½ tsp Salt
- 2/3 tsp Cumin
- Salsa:
- 1 Avocado, pitted and diced
- 1 Mango, diced
- 1 tbsp Olive Oil
- 1 tsp Honey
- ½ Red Onion, diced
- 2 tbsp Lime Juice
- Pinch of Salt

Directions:

1. Preheat your grill to 350-375 degrees F.
2. Place the olive oil and spices in a small bowl and rub the tuna steaks with the mixture.
3. Place on top of the bottom plate and cook for 4 minutes.
4. Flip the steaks over and cook for another 4 minutes.
5. Meanwhile, prepare the salsa by placing all of the salsa ingredients in a bowl, and mixing well to combine.
6. Transfer the grilled tuna steaks to two serving plates and divide the avocado and mango salsa among them.
7. Enjoy!

Nutrition Info: Calories 280 ;Total Fats 26g ;Carbs 12g ;Protein 24g ;Fiber: 2g

Blackened Tilapia

Servings: 4
Cooking Time: 8 Minutes

Ingredients:

- 4 Tilapia Fillets
- 3 tsp Paprika
- ½ tsp Garlic Powder
- ¼ tsp Onion Powder
- ¼ tsp Black Pepper
- ¾ tsp Salt
- 2 tbsp Olive Oil

Directions:

1. Preheat your grill to 375 degrees F.
2. Place the oil and spices in a small bowl and mix to combine.
3. Rub the mixture into the tilapia fillets, making sure to coat well.
4. When the green light indicates the unit is ready for grilling, arrange the tilapia onto the bottom plate.
5. With the lid off, cook for 4 minutes.
6. Flip over, and thencook for another four minutes. Feel free to increase the cooking time if you like your fish especially burnt.
7. Serve as desired and enjoy!

Nutrition Info: Calories 175 ;Total Fats 9g ;Carbs 1g ;Protein 23.5g ;Fiber: 0.6g

Shrimp Skewers

Servings: 4

Cooking Time: 4 Minutes

Ingredients:

- 1/3 cup lemon juice
- 2 tablespoons olive oil
- 2 garlic cloves, minced
- 1/2 teaspoon lemon zest, grated
- 1 lb. uncooked shrimp, peeled and deveined
- Salt and black pepper, to taste

Directions:

1. Season the shrimp with olive oil, salt, black pepper lemon juice, lemon zest, oil, and garlic in a suitable bowl.
2. Thread the seasoned shrimp on the skewers.
3. And season the skewers with salt and black pepper.
4. Turn the "Selector" knob to the "Grill Panini" side.
5. Preheat the bottom grill of Hamilton Beach Grill at 350 degrees F and the upper grill plate on medium heat.
6. Once it is preheated, open the lid and place the shrimp skewers in the Griddler.
7. Close the griddler's lid and grill the skewers for 4 minutes.
8. Serve warm.

Nutrition Info: (Per Serving): Calories 338 ;Total Fat 3.8 g ;Saturated Fat 0.7 g ;Cholesterol 22 mg ;Sodium 620 mg ;Total Carbs 28.3 g ;Fiber 2.4 g ;Sugar 1.2 g ;Protein 15.4 g

Soy Sauce Salmon

Servings: 4
Cooking Time: 10 Minutes

Ingredients:

- 2 tablespoons scallions, chopped
- ¾ teaspoon fresh ginger, minced
- 1 garlic clove, minced
- ½ teaspoon dried dill weed, crushed
- ¼ cup olive oil
- 2 tablespoons balsamic vinegar
- 2 tablespoons low-sodium soy sauce
- 4 (5-ounce) boneless salmon fillets

Directions:

1. Add all ingredients except for salmon in a large bowl and mix well.
2. Add salmon and coat with marinade generously.
3. Cover and refrigerate to marinate for at least 4-5 hours.
4. Place the water tray in the bottom of Hamilton Beach Grill.
5. Place about 2 cups of lukewarm water into the water tray.
6. Place the drip pan over water tray and then arrange the heating element.
7. Now, place the grilling pan over heating element.
8. Plugin the Hamilton Beach Grill and press the 'Power' button to turn it on.
9. Then press 'Fan" button.
10. Set the temperature settings according to manufacturer's directions.
11. Cover the grill with lid and let it preheat.
12. After preheating, remove the lid and grease the grilling pan.
13. Place the salmon fillets over the grilling pan.
14. Cover with the lid and cook for about 5 minutes per side.
15. Serve hot.

Nutrition Info: (Per Serving):Calories 303 ;Total Fat 21.4 g ;Saturated Fat 3.1 g ;Cholesterol 63 mg ;Sodium 504 mg ;Total Carbs 1.4 g ;Fiber 0.2 g ;Sugar 0.6 g ;Protein 28.2 g

Pistachio Pesto Shrimp

Servings: 4
Cooking Time: 4 Minutes

Ingredients:

- ¾ cup fresh arugula
- ½ cup fresh parsley, minced
- 1/3 cup shelled pistachios
- 2 tablespoons lemon juice
- 1 garlic clove, peeled
- ¼ teaspoon lemon zest, grated
- ½ cup olive oil
- ¼ cup Parmesan cheese, shredded
- ¼ teaspoon salt
- 1/8 teaspoon pepper
- 1 ½ lbs. jumbo shrimp, peeled and deveined

Directions:

1. Start by blending the arugula, parsley, pistachios, lemon juice, garlic, lemon zest, and olive oil in a blender until smooth.
2. Stir in salt, black pepper, Parmesan cheese, and mix well.
3. Toss the shrimp with the prepared sauce in a bowl then cover to refrigerate for 30 minutes.
4. Thread these pesto shrimps on the wooden skewers.
5. Turn the "Selector" knob to the "Grill Panini" side.
6. Preheat the bottom grill of Hamilton Beach Grill at 350 degrees F and the upper grill plate on medium heat.
7. Once it is preheated, open the lid and place the pesto skewers in the Griddler.
8. Close the griddler's lid and grill the shrimp skewers for 4 minutes.
9. Serve warm.

Nutrition Info: (Per Serving): Calories 293 ;Total Fat 16 g ;Saturated Fat 2.3 g ;Cholesterol 75 mg ;Sodium 386 mg ;Total Carbs 5.2 g ;Sugar 2.6 g ;Fiber 1.9 g ;Protein 34.2 g

BEEF, PORK & LAMB RECIPES

Lamb Kabobs

Servings: 6
Cooking Time: 10 Minutes

Ingredients:

- 1 large pineapple, cubed into 1½-inch size, divided
- 1 (½-inch) piece fresh ginger, chopped
- 2 garlic cloves, chopped
- Salt, as required
- 16-24-ounce lamb shoulder steak, trimmed and cubed into 1½-inch size
- Fresh mint leaves from a bunch
- Ground cinnamon, as required

Directions:

1. In a food processor, add about 1½ cups of pineapple, ginger, garlic and salt and pulse until smooth.
2. Transfer the mixture into a large bowl.
3. Add the chops and coat with mixture generously.
4. Refrigerate to marinate for about 1-2 hours.
5. Remove from the refrigerator.
6. Thread lamb cubes, remaining pineapple and mint leaves onto pre-soaked wooden skewers.
7. Place the water tray in the bottom of Hamilton Beach Grill.
8. Place about 2 cups of lukewarm water into the water tray.
9. Place the drip pan over water tray and then arrange the heating element.
10. Now, place the grilling pan over heating element.
11. Plugin the Hamilton Beach Grill and press the 'Power' button to turn it on.
12. Then press 'Fan" button.
13. Set the temperature settings according to manufacturer's directions.
14. Cover the grill with lid and let it preheat.
15. After preheating, remove the lid and grease the grilling pan.
16. Place the skewers over the grilling pan.
17. Cover with the lid and cook for about 10 minutes, turning occasionally.

Nutrition Info: (Per Serving):Calories 288 ;Total Fat 8.5 g ;Saturated Fat 3 g ;Cholesterol 102 mg ;Sodium 115 mg ;Total Carbs 20.2 g ;Fiber 2.1 g ;Sugar 14.9 g ;Protein 32.7 g

Glazed Pork Chops

Servings: 6
Cooking Time: 12 Minutes

Ingredients:

- 2 tablespoons fresh ginger root, minced
- 1 teaspoon garlic, minced
- 2 tablespoons fresh orange zest, grated finely
- ½ cup fresh orange juice
- 1 teaspoon garlic chile paste
- 2 tablespoons soy sauce
- Salt, as required
- 6 (½-inch thick) pork loin chops

Directions:

1. In a large bowl, mix together all ingredients except for chops.
2. Add chops and coat with marinade generously.
3. Cover and refrigerate to marinate for about 2 hours, tossing occasionally.
4. Place the water tray in the bottom of Hamilton Beach Grill.
5. Place about 2 cups of lukewarm water into the water tray.
6. Place the drip pan over water tray and then arrange the heating element.
7. Now, place the grilling pan over heating element.
8. Plugin the Hamilton Beach Grill and press the 'Power' button to turn it on.
9. Then press 'Fan" button.
10. Set the temperature settings according to manufacturer's directions.
11. Cover the grill with lid and let it preheat.
12. After preheating, remove the lid and grease the grilling pan.
13. Place the chops over the grilling pan.
14. Cover with the lid and cook for about 10-12 minutes, flipping once in the middle way or until desired doneness.
15. Serve hot.

Nutrition Info: (Per Serving):Calories 560 ;Total Fat 42.3 g ;Saturated Fat 15.9 g ;Cholesterol 146 mg ;Sodium 447 mg ;Total Carbs 3.5 g ;Fiber 0.3 g ;Sugar 1.9 g ;Protein 38.8 g

Lamb Steak

Servings: 6
Cooking Time: 4 Minutes
Ingredients:
- 2 garlic cloves, minced
- 2 tablespoons olive oil
- 2 teaspoons dried oregano, crushed
- 2 tablespoons sumac
- 2 teaspoons sweet paprika
- 12 lamb cutlets, trimmed

Directions:
1. In a bowl mix together all ingredients except for lamb cutlets.
2. Add the cutlets and coat with garlic mixture evenly.
3. Set aside for at least 10 minutes.
4. Place the water tray in the bottom of Hamilton Beach Grill.
5. Place about 2 cups of lukewarm water into the water tray.
6. Place the drip pan over water tray and then arrange the heating element.
7. Now, place the grilling pan over heating element.
8. Plugin the Hamilton Beach Grill and press the 'Power' button to turn it on.
9. Then press 'Fan" button.
10. Set the temperature settings according to manufacturer's directions.
11. Cover the grill with lid and let it preheat.
12. After preheating, remove the lid and grease the grilling pan.
13. Place the cutlets over the grilling pan.
14. Cover with the lid and cook for about 2 minutes from both sides or until desired doneness.
15. Serve hot.

Nutrition Info: (Per Serving):Calories 343 ;Total Fat 16.6 g ;Saturated Fat 4.9 g ;Cholesterol 144 mg ;Sodium 122 mg ;Total Carbs 1 g ;Fiber 0.5 g ;Sugar 0.1 g ;Protein 45.2 g

American Burger

Servings: 4

Cooking Time: 9 Minutes

Ingredients:

- 1/2 cup seasoned bread crumbs
- 1 large egg, lightly beaten
- 1/2 teaspoon salt
- 1/2 teaspoon pepper
- 1-lb. ground beef
- 1 tablespoon olive oil

Directions:

1. Take all the ingredients for a burger in a suitable bowl except the oil and the buns.
2. Mix them thoroughly together and make 4 of the ½ inch patties.
3. Brush these patties with olive oil.
4. Turn the "Selector" knob to the "Grill Panini" side.
5. Preheat the bottom grill of Hamilton Beach Grill at 350 degrees F and the upper grill plate on medium heat.
6. Once it is preheated, open the lid and place the patties in the Griddler.
7. Close the griddler's lid and grill the patties for 7-9 minutes.
8. Serve warm.

Nutrition Info: (Per Serving): Calories 301 ;Total Fat 15.8 g ;Saturated Fat 2.7 g ;Cholesterol 75 mg ;Sodium 389 mg ;Total Carbs 11.7 g ;Fiber 0.3g ;Sugar 0.1 g ;Protein 28.2 g

Grilled Lamb Chops

Servings: 6
Cooking Time: 18 Minutes

Ingredients:

- 2 large garlic cloves, crushed
- 1 tablespoon fresh rosemary leaves
- 1 teaspoon fresh thyme leaves
- Pinch cayenne pepper, to taste
- Sea salt, to taste
- 2 tablespoons olive oil
- 6 lamb chops, about 3/4-inch thick

Directions:

1. Rub the lamb chops with olive oil, garlic, rosemary, thyme, salt and cayenne pepper.
2. Cover the chops and marinate for 1-8 hours in the refrigerator.
3. Turn the "Selector" knob to the "Grill Panini" side.
4. Preheat the bottom grill of Hamilton Beach Grill at 350 degrees F and the upper grill plate on medium heat.
5. Once it is preheated, open the lid and place 3 chops in the Griddler.
6. Close the griddler's lid and grill the chops for 9 minutes.
7. Transfer them to a plate and grill the remaining chops in the same manner.
8. Serve warm.

Nutrition Info: (Per Serving): Calories 452 ;Total Fat 4 g ;Saturated Fat 2 g ;Cholesterol 65 mg ;Sodium 220 mg ;Total Carbs 23.1 g ;Fiber 0.3 g ;Sugar 1 g ;Protein 26g

Fajita Skewers

Servings: 6

Cooking Time: 7 Minutes

Ingredients:

- 1 lb. sirloin steak, cubed
- 1 bunch scallions, cut into large pieces
- 1 pack flour tortillas, cut into triangles
- 4 large bell peppers, cubed
- olive oil, for drizzling
- Salt to taste
- Black pepper to taste

Directions:

1. Thread the steak, tortillas, peppers, and scallions on the skewers.
2. Drizzle salt, black pepper, and olive oil over the skewers.
3. Turn the "Selector" knob to the "Grill Panini" side.
4. Preheat the bottom grill of Hamilton Beach Grill at 350 degrees F and the upper grill plate on medium heat.
5. Once it is preheated, open the lid and place the fajita skewers in the Griddler.
6. Close the griddler's lid and grill the skewers for 7 minutes.
7. Serve warm.

Nutrition Info: (Per Serving): Calories 353 ;Total Fat 7.5 g ;Saturated Fat 1.1 g ;Cholesterol 20 mg ;Sodium 297 mg ;Total Carbs 10.4 g ;Fiber 0.2 g ;Sugar 0.1 g ;Protein 13.1 g

Lamb Skewers

Servings: 6

Cooking Time: 10 Minutes

Ingredients:

- 1 (10 oz.) pack couscous
- 1 1/2 cup yogurt
- 1 tablespoon 1 teaspoon cumin
- 2 garlic cloves, minced
- Juice of 2 lemons
- Salt to taste
- Black pepper to taste
- 1 1/2 lb. leg of lamb, boneless, diced
- 2 tomatoes, diced
- 1/2 English cucumber, diced
- 1/2 small red onion, chopped
- 1/4 cup parsley, chopped
- 1/4 cup fresh mint, chopped
- 3 tablespoon olive oil

Directions:

1. First, cook the couscous as per the given instructions on the package then fluff with a fork.
2. Whisk yogurt with garlic, cumin, lemon juice, salt, and black pepper in a large bowl.
3. Add lamb and mix well to coat the meat.
4. Separately toss red onion with cucumber, tomatoes, parsley, mint, lemon juice, olive oil, salt, and couscous in salad bowl.
5. Thread the seasoned lamb on 8 skewers and drizzle salt and black pepper over them.
6. Turn the "Selector" knob to the "Grill Panini" side.
7. Preheat the bottom grill of Hamilton Beach Grill at 350 degrees F and the upper grill plate on medium heat.
8. Once it is preheated, open the lid and place the lamb skewers in the Griddler.
9. Close the griddler's lid and grill the lamb skewers for 10 minutes.
10. Serve warm with prepared couscous.

Nutrition Info: (Per Serving): Calories 472 ;Total Fat 11.1 g ;Saturated Fat 5.8 g ;Cholesterol 610 mg ;Sodium 749 mg ;Total Carbs 19.9 g ;Fiber 0.2 g ;Sugar 0.2 g ;Protein 13.5 g

Pork Burnt Ends

Servings: 1
Cooking Time: 6 Minutes
Ingredients:
- 1-pound Pork Shoulder
- 2 tbsp Favorite Rub Spice
- 2 tbsp Honey
- 1 ½ tbsp Barbecue Sauce

Directions:
1. Start by chopping the pork into cubes.
2. Place the meat in a bowl and add the spice, honey, and barbecue sauce.
3. With your hands, mix wel, making sure that each meat cube gets a little bit of honey, sauce, and spices.
4. Preheat your grill to 375 degrees F.
5. Arange the pork onto the bottom plate and lower the lid.
6. Cook for about 6 minutes.
7. Check the meat – if it is not too burnt for your taste, cook for an additional minute.
8. Serve as desired.
9. Enjoy!

Nutrition Info: Calories 399 ;Total Fats 27g ;Carbs 10.8g ;Protein 27g ;Fiber: 0g

Greek Souzoukaklia

Servings: 4
Cooking Time: 14 Minutes

Ingredients:

- 1 ½ pounds ground beef
- 1 onion, chopped
- ⅜ cup raisins, chopped
- 1 ½ teaspoons parsley, chopped
- ½ teaspoon cayenne pepper
- ½ teaspoon ground cinnamon
- ½ teaspoon ground coriander
- 1 pinch ground nutmeg
- ½ teaspoon white sugar
- Salt and black pepper to taste
- 1 tablespoon vegetable oil

Directions:

1. Mix ground beef with onion, raisins, and rest of the ingredients in a bowl.
2. Take a handful of this mixture and wrap it around each skewer to make a sausage.
3. Turn the "Selector" knob to the "Grill Panini" side.
4. Preheat the bottom grill of Hamilton Beach Grill at 350 degrees F and the upper grill plate on medium heat.
5. Once it is preheated, open the lid and place the skewers in the Griddler.
6. Close the griddler's lid and grill the skewers for 15 minutes.
7. Enjoy.

Nutrition Info: (Per Serving): Calories 361 ;Total Fat 16.3 g ;Saturated Fat 4.9 g ;Cholesterol 114 mg ;Sodium 515 mg ;Total Carbs 19.3 g ;Fiber 0.1 g ;Sugar 18.2 g ;Protein 33.3 g

Maple Pork Chops

Servings: 1

Cooking Time: 7-8 Minutes

Ingredients:

- 4 boneless Pork Chops
- 6 tbsp Balsamic Vinegar
- 6 tbsp Maple Syrup
- ¼ tsp ground Sage
- Salt and Pepper, to taste

Directions:

1. Whisk the vinegar, maple, sage, and some salt and pepper in a bowl.
2. Add the pork chops and coat well.
3. Cover with plastic foil and refrigerate for one hour.
4. Preheat your grill to 350 degrees F.
5. Open and arrange the chops onto the bottom plate.
6. Lower the lid and cook closed for about 7 minutes, or until your desired doneness is reached.
7. Serve and enjoy!

Nutrition Info: Calories 509 ;Total Fats 19g ;Carbs 15g ;Protein 65g ;Fiber: 0g

Sweet Ham Kabobs

Servings: 6

Cooking Time: 7 Minutes

Ingredients:

- 1 can (20 oz.) pineapple chunks
- 1/2 cup orange marmalade
- 1 tablespoon mustard
- ¼ teaspoon ground cloves
- 1 lb. ham, diced
- ½ lb. Swiss cheese, diced
- 1 medium green pepper, cubed

Directions:

1. Take 2 tablespoons of pineapple from pineapples in a bowl.
2. Add mustard, marmalade, and cloves mix well and keep it aside.
3. Thread the pineapple, green pepper, cheese, and ham over the skewers alternatively.
4. Turn the "Selector" knob to the "Grill Panini" side.
5. Preheat the bottom grill of Hamilton Beach Grill at 350 degrees F and the upper grill plate on medium heat.
6. Once it is preheated, open the lid and place the skewers in the Griddler.
7. Close the griddler's lid and grill the skewers for 7 minutes.
8. Serve warm with marmalade sauce on top.
9. Enjoy.

Nutrition Info: (Per Serving): Calories 301 ;Total Fat 8.9 g ;Saturated Fat 4.5 g ;Cholesterol 57 mg ;Sodium 340 mg ;Total Carbs 24.7 g ;Fiber 1.2 g ;Sugar 1.3 g ;Protein 15.3 g

Steak Skewers With Potatoes And Mushrooms

Servings: 6

Cooking Time: 10 Minutes

Ingredients:

- 1-pound Steak
- 4 tbsp Olive Oil
- ½ pound Button Mushrooms
- 4 tbsp Balsamic Vinegar
- 1 pound Very Small Potatoes, boiled
- 2 tsp minced Garlic
- ½ tsp dired Sage
- Salt and Pepper, to taste

Directions:

1. Start by cutting the steak into 1-inch pieces.
2. Quarter the mushrooms.
3. Whisk the vinegar, oil, garlic, sage, and salt and pepper, in a bowl.
4. Add the meat, murshooms and potatoes to the bowl, coat well, and place in the fridge for 30 minutes. If your potatoes are not small enough for the skewers, you can chop them into smaller chunks.
5. In the meantime, soak the skewers in cold water.
6. Meanwhile, preheat your grill to medium-high.
7. Thread the chunks onto the skewers and arrange them on the bottom plate.
8. Keep the lid open and cook for 5.
9. Flip over and cook for 5 more minutes.
10. Serve and enjoy!

Nutrition Info: Calories 383 ;Total Fats 23g ;Carbs 21g ;Protein 23g ;Fiber: 3g

Margarita Beef Skewers

Servings: 6
Cooking Time: 10 Minutes

Ingredients:

- 1 cup margarita mix
- ½ teaspoon salt
- 1 tablespoon white sugar
- 2 garlic cloves, minced
- ¼ cup vegetable oil
- 1-pound top sirloin steak, cubed
- 16 mushrooms, stems trimmed
- 1 onion, cut into chunks
- 1 large red bell pepper, diced

Directions:

1. Mix margarita, salt, white sugar, garlic, vegetable, sirloin steak, mushrooms, onion, and red bell pepper on a bowl.
2. Cover and refrigerate the beef mixture for 1 hour for marination.
3. Thread the beef, mushrooms, onion and bell pepper, alternately on the wooden.
4. Turn the "Selector" knob to the "Grill Panini" side.
5. Preheat the bottom grill of Hamilton Beach Grill at 350 degrees F and the upper grill plate on medium heat.
6. Once it is preheated, open the lid and place the skewers in the Griddler.
7. Close the griddler's lid and grill the skewers for 10 minutes.
8. Serve warm.

Nutrition Info: (Per Serving): Calories 405 ;Total Fat 22.7 g ;Saturated Fat 6.1 g ;Cholesterol 4 mg ;Sodium 227 mg ;Total Carbs 26.1 g ;Fiber 1.4 g ;Sugar 0.9 g ;Protein 45.2 g

Salisbury Steak

Servings: 5
Cooking Time: 12 Minutes

Ingredients:

- 1 1/2 pounds lean ground beef
- 1/2 cup seasoned breadcrumbs
- 1 tablespoon ketchup
- 2 teaspoons dry mustard
- 4 dashes Worcestershire sauce
- 1 cube beef bouillon, crumbled
- Salt and black pepper, to taste
- 1 tablespoon butter, melted

Directions:

1. Mix ground beef with breadcrumbs, ketchup, mustard, Worcestershire sauce, beef bouillon, butter, black pepper and salt in a bowl.
2. Make five patties out of the crumbly beef mixture.
3. Turn the "Selector" knob to the "Grill Panini" side.
4. Preheat the bottom grill of Hamilton Beach Grill at 350 degrees F and the upper grill plate on medium heat.
5. Once it is preheated, open the lid and place the patties in the Griddler.
6. Close the griddler's lid and grill the patties for 6 minutes.
7. Serve warm.

Nutrition Info: (Per Serving): Calories 548 ;Total Fat 22.9 g ;Saturated Fat 9 g ;Cholesterol 105 mg ;Sodium 350 mg ;Total Carbs 17.5 g ;Sugar 10.9 g ;Fiber 6.3 g ;Protein 40.1 g

Herbed Lemony Pork Skewers

Servings: 4

Cooking Time: 8 Minutes

Ingredients:

- 1-pound Pork Shoulder or Neck
- 1 tsp dried Basil
- 1 tsp dried Parsley
- 1 tsp dried Oregano
- 2 Garlic Cloves, minced
- 4 tbsp Lemon Juice
- ¼ tsp Onion Powder
- Salt and Pepper, to taste

Directions:

1. Start by soaking 8 skewers in cold water, to prevent the wood from burning on the grill.
2. Cut the pork into small chunks and place in a bowl.
3. Add lemon juice, garlic, spices and herbs to the bowl.
4. Give the mixture a good stir so that the meat is coated well.
5. Preheat your grill to medium-high.
6. Meanwhile, thread the meat onto the skewers.
7. When the green light turns on, arrange the skewers onto the bottom plate.
8. Cook for about 4 minutes per side (or more if you like the meat well-done and almost burnt).
9. Serve as desired and enjoy!

Nutrition Info: Calories 364 ;Total Fats 27g ;Carbs 1.6g ;Protein 26.7g ;Fiber: 0.1g

Rosemary Lamb Chops

Servings: 2

Cooking Time: 10 Minutes

Ingredients:

- 1 tablespoon olive oil
- 1 tablespoon fresh lemon juice
- 1 tablespoon fresh rosemary, chopped
- ½ teaspoon garlic, minced
- Salt and ground black pepper, as required
- 2 (8-ounce) (½-inch-thick) lamb shoulder blade chops

Directions:

1. In a bowl, place all ingredients and beat until well combined.
2. Place the chops and oat with the mixture well.
3. Seal the bag and shake vigorously to coat evenly.
4. Place the water tray in the bottom of Hamilton Beach Grill.
5. Place about 2 cups of lukewarm water into the water tray.
6. Place the drip pan over water tray and then arrange the heating element.
7. Now, place the grilling pan over heating element.
8. Plugin the Hamilton Beach Grill and press the 'Power' button to turn it on.
9. Then press 'Fan" button.
10. Set the temperature settings according to manufacturer's directions.
11. Cover the grill with lid and let it preheat.
12. After preheating, remove the lid and grease the grilling pan.
13. Place the lamb chops over the grilling pan.
14. Cover with the lid and cook for about 4-5 minutes per side.
15. Serve hot.

Nutrition Info: (Per Serving):Calories 410 ;Total Fat 25.4 g ;Saturated Fat 7.2 g ;Cholesterol 151 mg ;Sodium 241 mg ;Total Carbs 1.5 g ;Fiber 0.7 g ;Sugar 0.2 g ;Protein 44.3 g

Grilled Pork Chops

Servings: 4
Cooking Time: 20 Minutes
Ingredients:
- 4 pork chops bone in
- 1/4 cup olive oil
- 1 1/2 tablespoons brown sugar
- 2 teaspoons Dijon mustard
- 1 1/2 tablespoons soy sauce
- 1 teaspoon lemon zest
- 2 teaspoons parsley chopped
- 2 teaspoons thyme leaves, chopped
- 1/2 teaspoon salt
- 1/2 teaspoon black pepper
- 1 teaspoon garlic, minced

Directions:
1. Mix olive oil, brown sugar, Dijon mustard, soy sauce, lemon zest, parsley, thyme, salt, black pepper and garlic in a large and shallow bowl.
2. Add pork chops to the mixture and rub the spices all over.
3. Cover the pork chops and refrigerate for 1-8 hours for marination.
4. Turn the "Selector" knob to the "Grill Panini" side.
5. Preheat the bottom grill of Hamilton Beach Grill at 350 degrees F and the upper grill plate on medium heat.
6. Once it is preheated, open the lid and place 2 pork chops in the Griddler.
7. Close the griddler's lid and grill the pork chops for 10 minutes.
8. Cook the rest of the chops in the same way.
9. Serve warm.

Nutrition Info: (Per Serving): Calories 545 ;Total Fat 36.4 g ;Saturated Fat 10.1 g ;Cholesterol 200 mg ;Sodium 272 mg ;Total Carbs 40.7 g ;Fiber 0.2 g ;Sugar 0.1 g ;Protein 42.5 g

Spiced Lamb Chops

Servings: 8
Cooking Time: 8 Minutes

Ingredients:

- 1 tablespoon fresh mint leaves, chopped
- 1 teaspoon garlic paste
- 1 teaspoon ground allspice
- ½ teaspoon ground nutmeg
- ½ teaspoon ground green cardamom
- ¼ teaspoon hot paprika
- Salt and ground black pepper, as required
- 4 tablespoons olive oil
- 2 tablespoons fresh lemon juice
- 2 racks of lamb, trimmed and separated into 16 chops

Directions:

1. In a large bowl, add all the ingredients except for chops and mix until well combined.
2. Add the chops and coat with the mixture generously.
3. Refrigerate to marinate for about 5-6 hours.
4. Place the water tray in the bottom of Hamilton Beach Grill.
5. Place about 2 cups of lukewarm water into the water tray.
6. Place the drip pan over water tray and then arrange the heating element.
7. Now, place the grilling pan over heating element.
8. Plugin the Hamilton Beach Grill and press the 'Power' button to turn it on.
9. Then press 'Fan" button.
10. Set the temperature settings according to manufacturer's directions.
11. Cover the grill with lid and let it preheat.
12. After preheating, remove the lid and grease the grilling pan.
13. Place the lamb chops over the grilling pan.
14. Cover with the lid and cook for about 6-8 minutes, flipping once halfway through.
15. Serve hot.

Nutrition Info: (Per Serving):Calories 380 ;Total Fat 19.6 g ;Saturated Fat 5.6 g ;Cholesterol 153 mg ;Sodium 150 mg ;Total Carbs 0.5 g ;Fiber 0.2 g ;Sugar 0.1 g ;Protein 47.9 g

Garlicky Marinated Steak

Servings: 1

Cooking Time: 8 Minutes

Ingredients:

- 4 Steaks (about 1 - 1 ½ pounds)
- 3 tbsp minced Garlic
- ¼ cup Soy Sauce
- 2 tbsp Honey
- ¼ cup Balsamic Vinegar
- 2 tbsp Worcesteshire Sauce
- ½ tsp Onion Powder
- Salt and Pepper, to taste

Directions:

1. Whisk together the garlic, sauces, and spices, in a bowl.
2. Add the steaks to it and make sure to coat them well.
3. Cover with plastic foil and refrigerate for about an hour.
4. Preheat your grill to high.
5. Open and add your steaks to the bottom plate.
6. Lower the lid and cook for about 4 minutes, or until the meat reaches the internal temperature that you prefer.
7. Serve as desired and let sit for a couple of minutes before enjoying!

Nutrition Info: Calories 435 ;Total Fats 24g ;Carbs 19g ;Protein 37g ;Fiber: 1g

Spicy Pork Chops

Servings: 4
Cooking Time: 15 Minutes

Ingredients:

- 2 teaspoons Worcestershire sauce
- 1 teaspoon liquid smoke flavoring
- 1 tablespoon onion powder
- 1 tablespoon garlic powder
- 1 tablespoon paprika
- 1 tablespoon seasoned salt
- 1 teaspoon freshly ground black pepper
- 4 (½-¾-inch thick) bone-in pork chops

Directions:

1. In a bowl, mix together all ingredients except for chops.
2. Add chops and coat with mixture generously.
3. Set aside for about 10-15 minutes.
4. Place the water tray in the bottom of Hamilton Beach Grill.
5. Place about 2 cups of lukewarm water into the water tray.
6. Place the drip pan over water tray and then arrange the heating element.
7. Now, place the grilling pan over heating element.
8. Plugin the Hamilton Beach Grill and press the 'Power' button to turn it on.
9. Then press 'Fan" button.
10. Set the temperature settings according to manufacturer's directions.
11. Cover the grill with lid and let it preheat.
12. After preheating, remove the lid and grease the grilling pan.
13. Place the chops over the grilling pan.
14. Cover with the lid and cook for about 15 minutes, flipping once halfway through.
15. Serve hot.

Nutrition Info: (Per Serving):Calories 262 ;Total Fat 12.3 g ;Saturated Fat 4.1 g ;Cholesterol 85 mg ;Sodium 1800 mg ;Total Carbs 5.7 g ;Fiber 1.1 g ;Sugar 2.8 g ;Protein 29.9 g

SNACK & DESSERT RECIPES

Nectarine

Servings: 2
Cooking Time: 6 Minutes
Ingredients:
- 2 medium nectarines, halved and pitted
- 1 tablespoon butter, melted
- 2 tablespoons honey
- ½ teaspoon ground nutmeg

Directions:
1. Brush the nectarine halves with butter evenly.
2. Place the water tray in the bottom of Hamilton Beach Grill.
3. Place about 2 cups of lukewarm water into the water tray.
4. Place the drip pan over water tray and then arrange the heating element.
5. Now, place the grilling pan over heating element.
6. Plugin the Hamilton Beach Grill and press the 'Power' button to turn it on.
7. Then press 'Fan" button.
8. Set the temperature settings according to manufacturer's directions.
9. Cover the grill with lid and let it preheat.
10. After preheating, remove the lid and grease the grilling pan.
11. Place the nectarine halves over the grilling pan.
12. Cook, uncovered for about 5-6 minutes, flipping and brushing with honey occasionally.
13. Transfer the nectarine halves onto a platter and set aside to cool.
14. Sprinkle with nutmeg and serve.

Nutrition Info: (Per Serving):Calories 180 ;Total Fat 6.4 g ;Saturated Fat 3.8 g ;Cholesterol 15 mg ;Sodium 42 mg ;Total Carbs 32.6 g ;Fiber 2.6 g ;Sugar 28.6 g ;Protein 1.7 g

Blueberry Waffles

Servings: 4
Cooking Time: 6 Minutes

Ingredients:

- ¼ cup all-purpose flour
- 1 teaspoon baking powder
- 2 tablespoons butter, melted
- 2 large eggs
- 2 ounces blueberry preserves
- ¼ cup powdered sugar
- 1½ teaspoons vanilla extract

Directions:

1. Turn the "Selector" knob to the "Grill Panini" side.
2. Fix a waffle plates in the cuisine gr Griddler, preheat it at 350 degrees F and preheat the upper plate on medium heat.
3. In a bowl, add the butter and eggs and beat until creamy.
4. Add the blueberry preserves, sugar, vanilla extract and salt and beat until well combined.
5. Add the flour and baking powder and beat until well combined.
6. Pour ¼ of the mixture into preheated Griddler, close the lid and cook for about 3 minutes.
7. Cook for waffle using the remaining batter.
8. Serve warm.

Nutrition Info: (Per Serving): Calories 215 ;Total Fat 8.5 g ;Saturated Fat 9.1 g ;Cholesterol 116 mg ;Sodium 131 mg ;Total Carbs 21.6 g ;Fiber 1.1 g ;Sugar 4.7 g ;Protein 3.8 g

Double Chocolate Pancakes

Servings: 2
Cooking Time: 4 Minutes
Ingredients:

- 2 teaspoons coconut flour
- 2 tablespoons sugar
- 1 tablespoon cacao powder
- ¼ teaspoon baking powder
- 1 egg
- 1-ounce cream cheese, softened
- ½ teaspoon vanilla extract
- 1 tablespoon 70% dark chocolate chips

Directions:

1. Turn the "Selector" knob to the "Griddle" side.
2. Preheat the bottom plate of the Cuisine GR Griddler at 350 degrees F.
3. In a bowl, add flour, Sugar, cacao powder and baking powder and mix well.
4. Add the egg, cream cheese and vanilla extract and beat until well combined.
5. Gently, fold in the chocolate chips.
6. Pour ½ of the mixture into preheated Griddler and cook for about 2 minutes per side.
7. Cook more pancakes using the remaining batter.
8. Serve warm.

Nutrition Info: (Per Serving): Calories 151 ;Total Fat 11.9 g ;Saturated Fat 6.8 g ;Cholesterol 97 mg ;Sodium 76 mg ;Total Carbs 15.9 g ;Fiber 2.8 g ;Sugar 0.3 g ;Protein 5.7 g

Chocolate-covered Grilled Strawberries

Servings: 4

Cooking Time: 6 Minutes

Ingredients:

- 12 Large Strawberries
- 3 ounces Chocolate
- 1 tbsp Butter

Directions:

1. Preheat your grill to 350 degrees F.
2. Clean and hull the strawberries.
3. When the green light appears, arrange the strawberries onto the plate.
4. Grill for about 6 minutes, rotating occasionally for even cooking.
5. Melt the chocolate and butter in a microwave. Stir to combine.
6. Coat the grilled strawberries with the melted chocolate and arrange on a platter.
7. Let harden before consuming.
8. Enjoy!

Nutrition Info: Calories 146 ;Total Fats 8g ;Carbs 18.3g ;Protein 1.4g ;Fiber: 1.6g

Pineapple

Servings: 6
Cooking Time: 10 Minutes

Ingredients:

- ¾ cup tequila
- ¾ cup brown sugar
- 1½ teaspoons vanilla extract
- ½ teaspoon ground cinnamon
- 1 large pineapple, peeled, cored and cut into 1-inch-thick slices

Directions:

1. Place tequila, sugar, vanilla and cinnamon in a bowl and mix well.
2. Place the water tray in the bottom of Hamilton Beach Grill.
3. Place about 2 cups of lukewarm water into the water tray.
4. Place the drip pan over water tray and then arrange the heating element.
5. Now, place the grilling pan over heating element.
6. Plugin the Hamilton Beach Grill and press the 'Power' button to turn it on.
7. Then press 'Fan" button.
8. Set the temperature settings according to manufacturer's directions.
9. Cover the grill with lid and let it preheat.
10. After preheating, remove the lid and grease the grilling pan.
11. Place the pineapple slices over the grilling pan.
12. Cover with the lid and cook for about 10 minutes, flipping and basting with tequila mixture occasionally.
13. Serve hot.

Nutrition Info: (Per Serving):Calories 225 ;Total Fat 0.2 g ;Saturated Fat 0 g ;Cholesterol 0 mg ;Sodium 8 mg ;Total Carbs 38.3 g ;Fiber 2.2 g ;Sugar 33 g ;Protein 0.8 g

Red Velvet Pancakes

Servings: 2

Cooking Time: 4 Minutes

Ingredients:

- 2 tablespoons cacao powder
- 2 tablespoons Sugar
- 1 egg, beaten
- 2 drops super red food coloring
- ¼ teaspoon baking powder
- 1 tablespoon heavy whipping cream

Directions:

1. Turn the "Selector" knob to the "Griddle" side.
2. Preheat the bottom plate of the Cuisine GR Griddler at 350 degrees F.
3. In a medium bowl, put all ingredients and with a fork, mix until well combined.
4. Pour ½ of the mixture into preheated Griddler and cook for about 2 minutes per side.
5. Cook more pancakes using the remaining batter.
6. Serve warm.

Nutrition Info: (Per Serving): Calories 370 ;Total Fat 6 g ;Saturated Fat 3 g ;Cholesterol 92 mg ;Sodium 34 mg ;Total Carbs 33.2 g ;Fiber 1.5 g ;Sugar 0.2 g ;Protein 3.9 g

Grilled Tomatoes With Garlic & Parmesan

Servings: 8

Cooking Time: 6 Minutes

Ingredients:

- ½ cup grated Parmesan Cheese
- 8 small Tomatoes, halved
- 1 tsp Garlic Powder
- 2 tbsp Olive Oil
- ¼ tsp Onion Powder
- Salt and Pepper, to taste

Directions:

1. Preheat your grill to 350 degrees F.
2. Combine the oil, garlic powder, onion powder, and salt and pepper, in a bowl.
3. Brush the tomatoes with this mixture.
4. Open the grill and arrange the tomatoes onto the plate.
5. Cook for 3 minutes, then flip over and cook for 2 more minutes.
6. Top with the parmesan cheese and cook for an additional minute.
7. Serve and enjoy!

Nutrition Info: Calories 78 ;Total Fats 5.6g ;Carbs 4.5g ;Protein 3.4g ;Fiber: 1g

Apple Crips In Foil

Servings: 8
Cooking Time: 20 Minutes

Ingredients:

- 4 Apples, sliced
- ½ cup Flour
- 4 tbsp Sugar
- 2 tsp Cinnamon
- ½ cup Quick Oats
- ½ cup Butter, melted
- ½ cup Brown Sugar
- ½ tsp Baking Powder

Directions:

1. Preheat your grill to 350 degrees F.
2. Prepare 4 aluminium foil squares (about 8x12 inches each).
3. Divide the apple slices among the foil and sprinkle with sugar and cinnamon.
4. In a bowl, combine the remaining ingredients well.
5. Divide the mixture evenly among the foil packets.
6. Carefully foil the packets, sealing so the filling stays inside.
7. When ready, open the grill and unlock the hinge.
8. Lay the griddle grate on top of your counter and place the foils there.
9. Cook for about 10 minutes.
10. Then, flip over, and cook for 10 minutes more.
11. Carefully open the packets and let sit for about 10 minutes before consuming.
12. Enjoy!

Nutrition Info: Calories 318 ;Total Fats 7g ;Carbs 51g ;Protein 2g ;Fiber: 3g

Banana Butter Kabobs

Servings: 6

Cooking Time: 3 Minutes

Ingredients:

- 1 loaf (10 ¾ oz.) cake, cubed
- 2 large bananas, one-inch slices
- 1/4 cup butter, melted
- 2 tablespoons brown sugar
- 1/2 teaspoon vanilla extract
- 1/8 teaspoon ground cinnamon
- 4 cups butter pecan ice cream
- 1/2 cup butterscotch ice cream topping
- 1/2 cup pecans, chopped and toasted

Directions:

1. Thread the cake and bananas over the skewers alternately.
2. Whisk butter with cinnamon, vanilla, and brown sugar in a small bowl.
3. Brush this mixture over the skewers liberally.
4. Turn the "Selector" knob to the "Grill Panini" side.
5. Preheat the bottom grill of Hamilton Beach Grill at 300 degrees F and the upper grill plate on medium heat.
6. Once it is preheated, open the lid and place the banana skewers in the Griddler.
7. Close the griddler's lid and grill the skewers for 3 minutes.
8. Serve with ice cream, pecan, and butterscotch topping on top.

Nutrition Info: (Per Serving): Calories 419 ;Total Fat 19.7 g ;Saturated Fat 18.6 g ;Cholesterol 141 mg ;Sodium 193 mg ;Total Carbs 23.7 g ;Fiber 0.9 g ;Sugar 19.3 g ;Protein 5.2 g

Grilled Melon With Honey & Lime

Servings: 4
Cooking Time: 6 Minutes

Ingredients:

- ½ small Melon
- 2 tbsp Honey
- Juice of 1 Lime
- Pinch of Salt
- Pinch of Pepper

Directions:

1. Preheat your grill to medium high.
2. In the meantime, peel the melon and cut into wedges.
3. When the green light appears, open the grill and coat with cooking spray.
4. Arrange the melon wedges onto the bottom plate of your HB grill.
5. Cook for about 3 minutes.
6. Flip over and cook for another three minutes.
7. Whisk together the honey, lime, salt, and pepper, and brush the grilled melon with this mixture.
8. Serve and enjoy!

Nutrition Info: Calories 92 ;Total Fats 2g ;Carbs 24g ;Protein 2g ;Fiber: 4g

Raspberry Pancakes

Servings: 2

Cooking Time: 4 Minutes

Ingredients:

- 1 egg, beaten
- 1 tablespoon cream cheese, softened
- ½ cup Mozzarella cheese, shredded
- 1 tablespoon powdered sugar
- ¼ teaspoon raspberry extract
- ¼ teaspoon vanilla extract

Directions:

1. Turn the "Selector" knob to the "Griddle" side.
2. Preheat the bottom plate of the Cuisine GR Griddler at 350 degrees F.
3. In a medium bowl, put all ingredients and with a fork, mix until well combined.
4. Pour ½ of the mixture into preheated Griddler and cook for about 2 minutes per side.
5. Cook more pancakes using the remaining batter.
6. Serve warm.

Nutrition Info: (Per Serving): Calories 269 ;Total Fat 5.2 g ;Saturated Fat 2.5 g ;Cholesterol 91 mg ;Sodium 88 mg ;Total Carbs 30.6 g ;Fiber 0 g ;Sugar 0.2 g ;Protein 5.2 g

Cinnamon Pancakes

Servings: 2
Cooking Time: 4 Minutes

Ingredients:

- 1 large egg, beaten
- ¾ cup mozzarella cheese, shredded
- ½ tablespoon unsalted butter, melted
- 2 tablespoons all-purpose flour
- 2 tablespoons sugar
- ½ teaspoon ground cinnamon
- ½ teaspoon psyllium husk powder
- ¼ teaspoon baking powder
- ½ teaspoon vanilla extract
- For Topping:
- 1 teaspoon powdered sugar
- ¾ teaspoon ground cinnamon

Directions:

1. Turn the "Selector" knob to the "Griddle" side.
2. Preheat the bottom plate of the Cuisine GR Griddler at 350 degrees F.
3. In a medium bowl, put all ingredients and with a fork, mix until well combined.
4. Pour ¼ of the mixture into preheated Griddler and cook for about 2 minutes per side.
5. Cook more pancakes using the remaining batter.
6. Meanwhile, for topping: in a small bowl, mix together the sugar and cinnamon.
7. Place the pancakes onto serving plates and set aside to cool slightly.
8. Sprinkle with the cinnamon mixture and serve immediately.

Nutrition Info: (Per Serving): Calories 242 ;Total Fat 10.6 g ;Saturated Fat 4 g ;Cholesterol 106 mg ;Sodium 122 mg ;Total Carbs 24.1 g ;Fiber 2 g ;Sugar 0.3 g ;Protein 7.7 g

CPSIA information can be obtained
at www.ICGtesting.com
Printed in the USA
LVHW020519070121
675853LV00018B/1149